THE **STUDENT'S MANUAL OF**

Yoga Anatomy

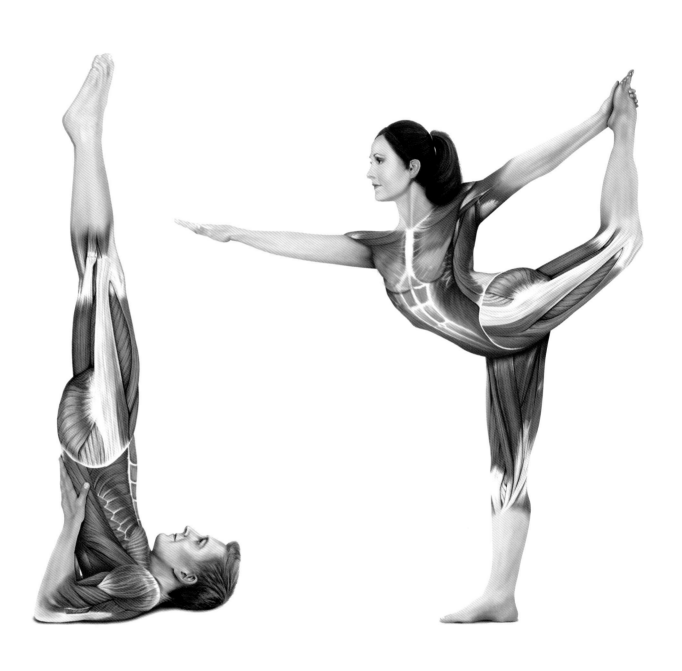

THE **STUDENT'S MANUAL OF**

Yoga Anatomy

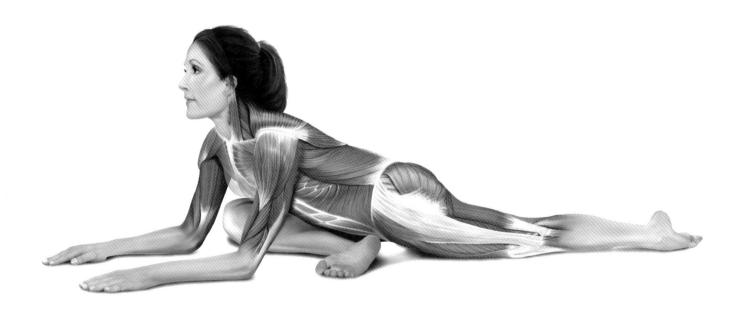

FAIR WINDS

Sally Parkes Bsc

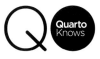

Quarto is the authority on a wide range of topics.

Quarto educates, entertains and enriches the lives of our readers—enthusiasts and lovers of hands-on living.

www.QuartoKnows.com

First published in the United States of America in 2016 by
Fair Winds Press, an imprint of
Quarto Publishing Group USA Inc.
100 Cummings Center
Suite 406-L
Beverly, Massachusetts 01915-6101
Telephone: (978) 282-9590
Fax: (978) 283-2742
QuartoKnows.com
Visit our blogs at QuartoKnows.com

20 19 18 17 16   1 2 3 4 5

ISBN: 978-1-59233-731-6

Design: Mike LeBihan
Cover Images: Joanna Culley, B.A. (Hons), R.M.I.P., M.M.M.A.,
medical-artist.com

Illustrations (Asana): Joanna Culley, B.A., (Hons), R.M.I.P., M.M.M.A.,
medical-artist.com

Illustrations (Steps): Robert Brandt

Other Illustrations:
David Carroll, Peter Child, Deborah Clarke, Geoff Cook, Marcus Cremonese, Beth Croce, Hans De Haas, Wendy de Paauw, Levant Efe, Mike Golding, Mike Gorman, Jeff Lang, Alex Lavroff, Ulrich Lehmann, Ruth Lindsay, Richard McKenna, Annabel Milne, Tony Pyrzakowski, Oliver Rennert, Caroline Rodrigues, Otto Schmidinger, Bob Seal, Vicky Short, Graeme Tavendale, Thomson Digital, Jonathan Tidball, Paul Tresnan, Valentin Varetsa, Glen Vause, Spike Wademan, Trevor Weekes, Paul Williams, David Wood

Printed in China

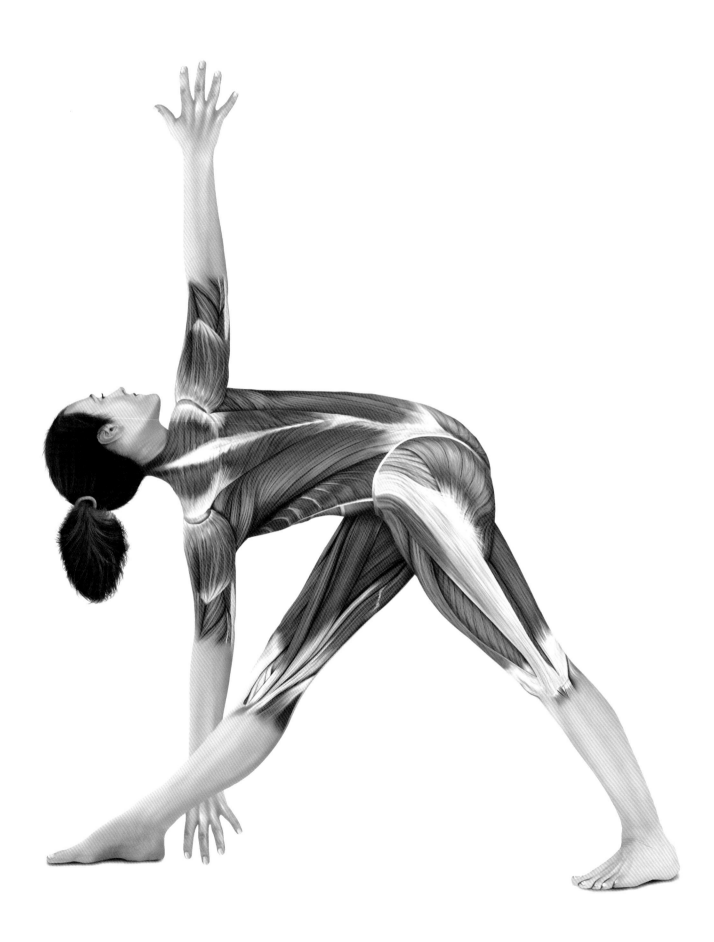

Contents

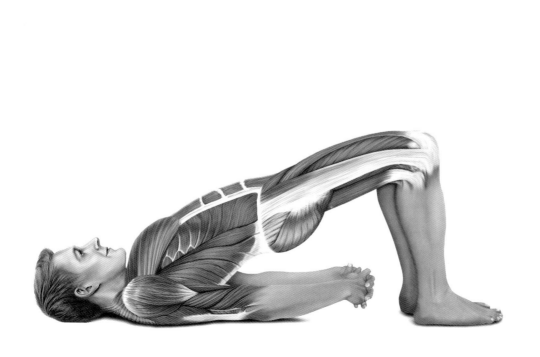

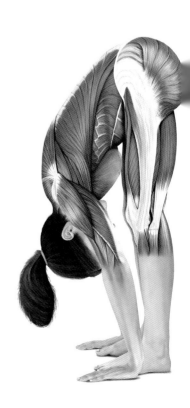

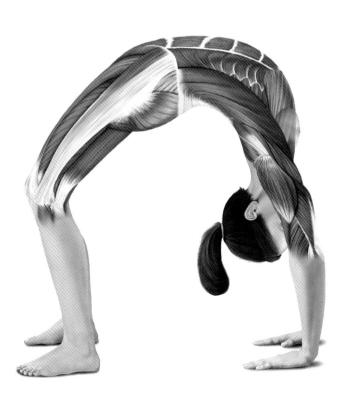

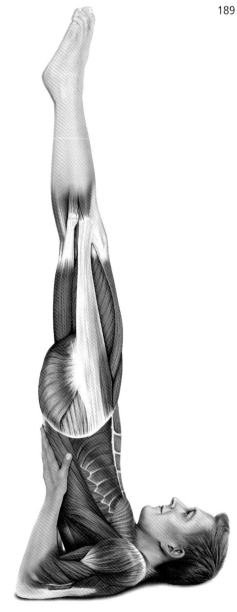

How This Book Works

This book is organized into three primary sections: a full-color anatomy overview; a principles of yoga section; and a full-color illustrated guide to thirty yoga asanas, or postures, comprising the main part of the book.

The Anatomy Overview section provides detailed, anatomically correct illustrations with clear, informative labels for the various body systems and regions.

The Principles of Yoga section examines the origins, history, and effects of the practice of yoga, and introduces some common yoga props and the four recurring starting positions that are referenced throughout the book.

The main content examining thirty yoga asanas is split into six chapters that divide the asanas into types: standing poses, standing balancing poses, standing forward bends, sitting poses, backbending poses, and inversions.

Each yoga asana has four pages of explanation. The first two pages introduce the asana, summarizing its benefits and origins, and offer tips on how to get the most out of it (and also advises what not to do). There are also clear step-by-step instructions and simple illustrations to help you achieve the correct posture.

The second two-page spread for each asana contains the more technical anatomical information. A brief summary discusses the main muscle activity in the asana, a clear table lists the main active muscles (and the type of activity), and stunning full-color anatomical illustrations are labeled to show the key muscles during the pose.

The book concludes with four pages of suggested sequences, allowing you to combine the asana into flowing movements.

ANATOMY OVERVIEW PAGES

This section contains full-color, double-page overview spreads that give a rundown of the important parts of a particular body system.

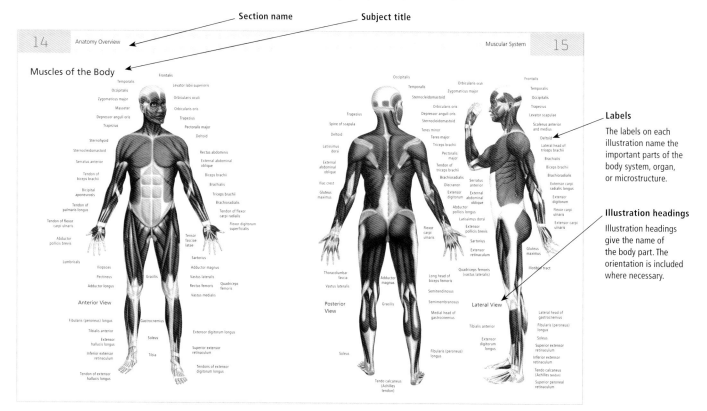

ASANA STEP-BY-STEP PAGES

Chapter name   Asana name

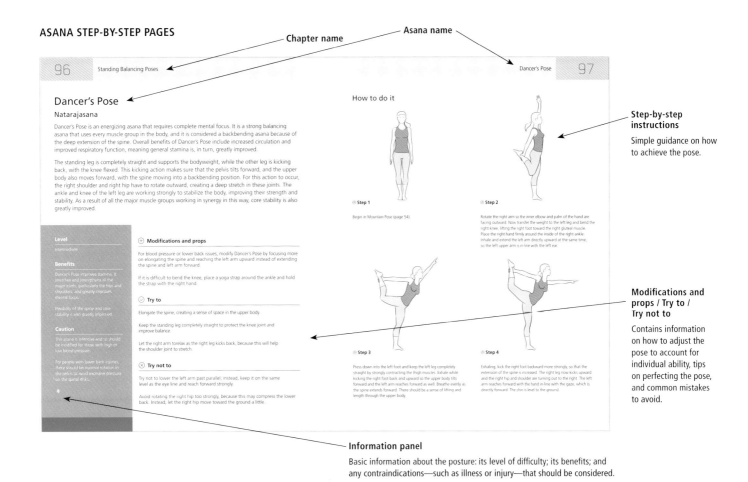

Step-by-step instructions
Simple guidance on how to achieve the pose.

Modifications and props / Try to / Try not to
Contains information on how to adjust the pose to account for individual ability, tips on perfecting the pose, and common mistakes to avoid.

Information panel
Basic information about the posture: its level of difficulty; its benefits; and any contraindications—such as illness or injury—that should be considered.

ASANA ANATOMY PAGES

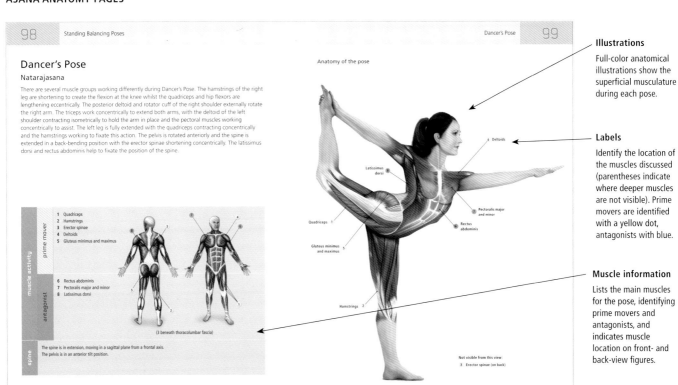

Illustrations
Full-color anatomical illustrations show the superficial musculature during each pose.

Labels
Identify the location of the muscles discussed (parentheses indicate where deeper muscles are not visible). Prime movers are identified with a yellow dot, antagonists with blue.

Muscle information
Lists the main muscles for the pose, identifying prime movers and antagonists, and indicates muscle location on front- and back-view figures.

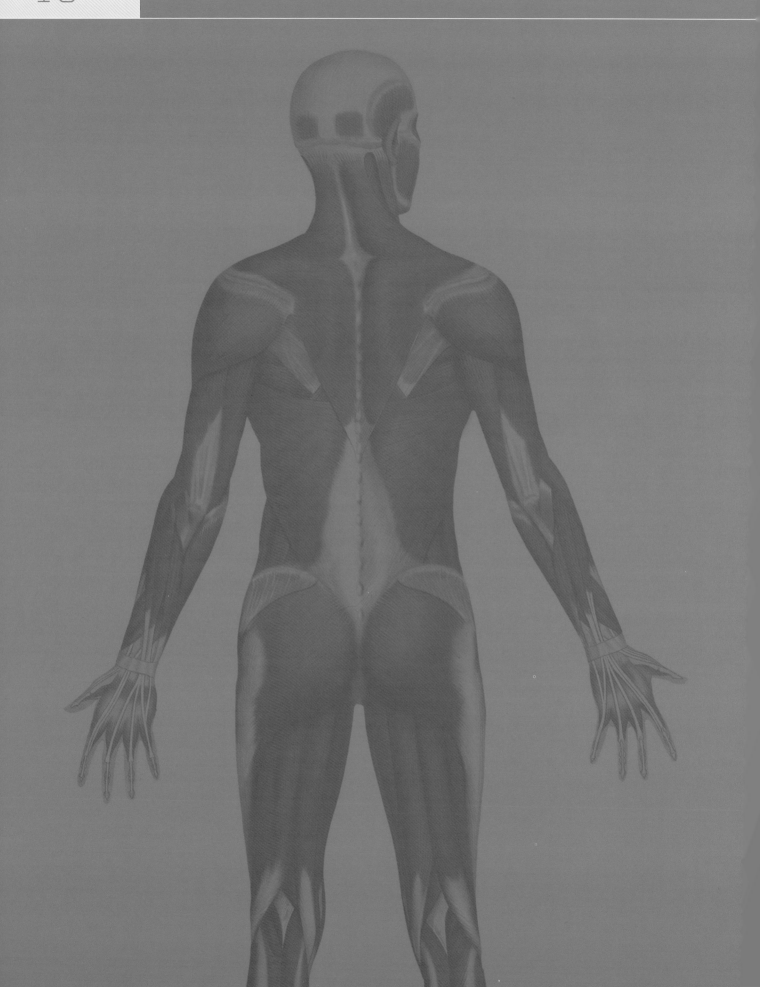

Anatomy Overview

Body Regions

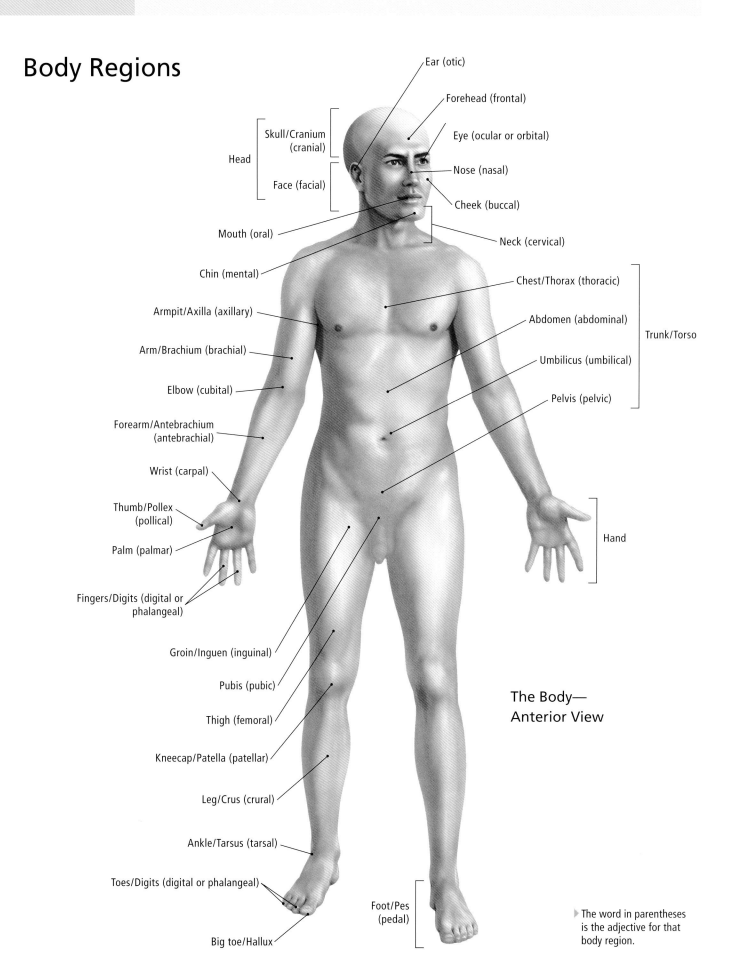

Ear (otic)

Forehead (frontal)

Eye (ocular or orbital)

Skull/Cranium (cranial)

Head

Face (facial)

Nose (nasal)

Cheek (buccal)

Mouth (oral)

Neck (cervical)

Chin (mental)

Chest/Thorax (thoracic)

Armpit/Axilla (axillary)

Abdomen (abdominal)

Arm/Brachium (brachial)

Umbilicus (umbilical)

Trunk/Torso

Elbow (cubital)

Pelvis (pelvic)

Forearm/Antebrachium (antebrachial)

Wrist (carpal)

Thumb/Pollex (pollical)

Palm (palmar)

Hand

Fingers/Digits (digital or phalangeal)

Groin/Inguen (inguinal)

Pubis (pubic)

The Body—
Anterior View

Thigh (femoral)

Kneecap/Patella (patellar)

Leg/Crus (crural)

Ankle/Tarsus (tarsal)

Toes/Digits (digital or phalangeal)

Foot/Pes (pedal)

Big toe/Hallux

▶ The word in parentheses is the adjective for that body region.

The Body—
Posterior View

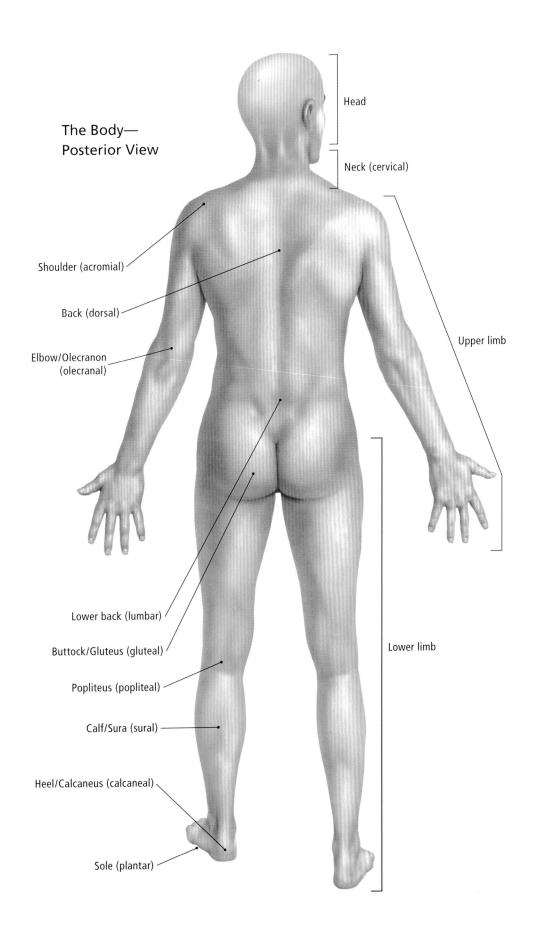

Head

Neck (cervical)

Shoulder (acromial)

Back (dorsal)

Elbow/Olecranon
(olecranal)

Upper limb

Lower back (lumbar)

Buttock/Gluteus (gluteal)

Popliteus (popliteal)

Calf/Sura (sural)

Heel/Calcaneus (calcaneal)

Sole (plantar)

Lower limb

Muscles of the Body

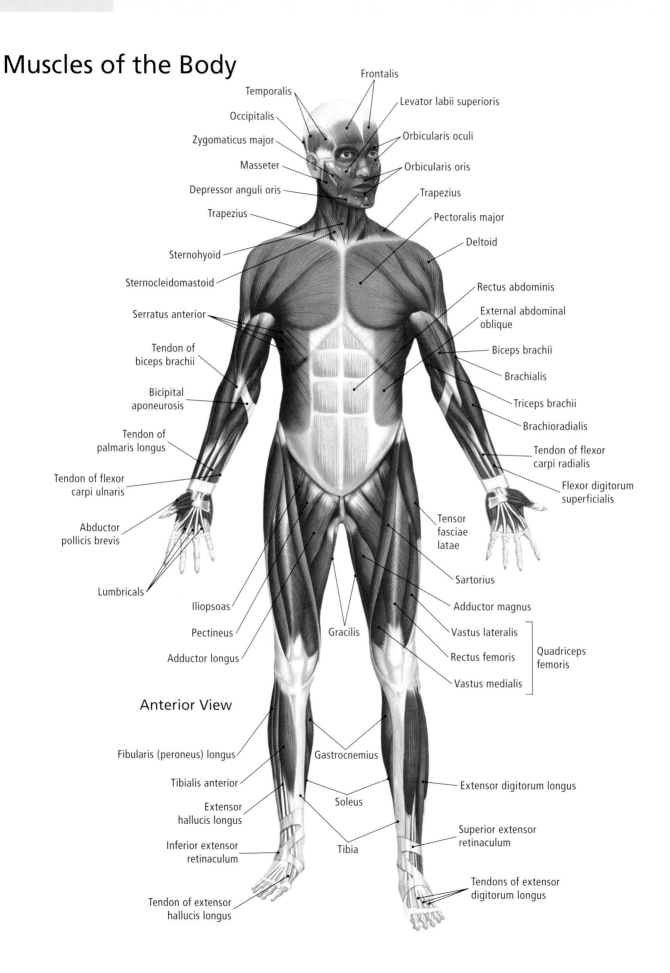

Temporalis

Occipitalis

Zygomaticus major

Masseter

Depressor anguli oris

Trapezius

Sternohyoid

Sternocleidomastoid

Serratus anterior

Tendon of
biceps brachii

Bicipital
aponeurosis

Tendon of
palmaris longus

Tendon of flexor
carpi ulnaris

Abductor
pollicis brevis

Lumbricals

Iliopsoas

Pectineus

Adductor longus

Anterior View

Fibularis (peroneus) longus

Tibialis anterior

Extensor
hallucis longus

Inferior extensor
retinaculum

Tendon of extensor
hallucis longus

Frontalis

Levator labii superioris

Orbicularis oculi

Orbicularis oris

Trapezius

Pectoralis major

Deltoid

Rectus abdominis

External abdominal
oblique

Biceps brachii

Brachialis

Triceps brachii

Brachioradialis

Tendon of flexor
carpi radialis

Flexor digitorum
superficialis

Tensor
fasciae
latae

Sartorius

Adductor magnus

Vastus lateralis

Rectus femoris

Vastus medialis

Quadriceps
femoris

Gracilis

Gastrocnemius

Soleus

Tibia

Extensor digitorum longus

Superior extensor
retinaculum

Tendons of extensor
digitorum longus

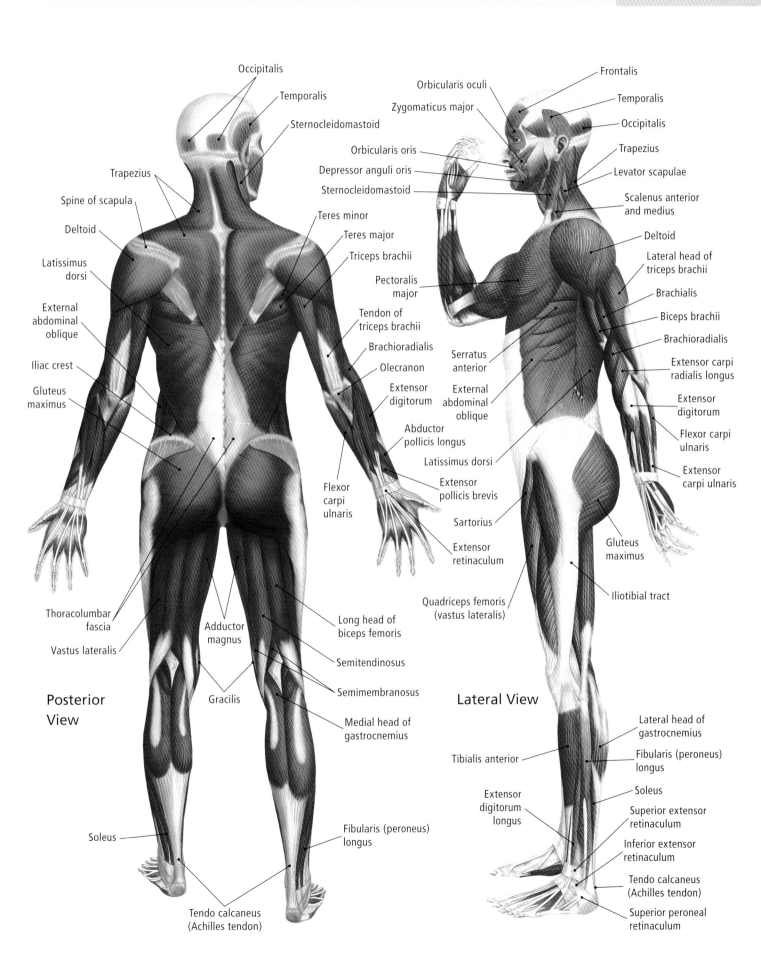

Posterior View

- Occipitalis
- Temporalis
- Sternocleidomastoid
- Trapezius
- Spine of scapula
- Deltoid
- Latissimus dorsi
- External abdominal oblique
- Iliac crest
- Gluteus maximus
- Teres minor
- Teres major
- Triceps brachii
- Tendon of triceps brachii
- Brachioradialis
- Olecranon
- Extensor digitorum
- Abductor pollicis longus
- Flexor carpi ulnaris
- Thoracolumbar fascia
- Vastus lateralis
- Adductor magnus
- Gracilis
- Long head of biceps femoris
- Semitendinosus
- Semimembranosus
- Medial head of gastrocnemius
- Soleus
- Fibularis (peroneus) longus
- Tendo calcaneus (Achilles tendon)

Lateral View

- Frontalis
- Orbicularis oculi
- Zygomaticus major
- Orbicularis oris
- Depressor anguli oris
- Sternocleidomastoid
- Temporalis
- Occipitalis
- Trapezius
- Levator scapulae
- Scalenus anterior and medius
- Deltoid
- Lateral head of triceps brachii
- Brachialis
- Biceps brachii
- Brachioradialis
- Extensor carpi radialis longus
- Extensor digitorum
- Flexor carpi ulnaris
- Extensor carpi ulnaris
- Pectoralis major
- Serratus anterior
- External abdominal oblique
- Latissimus dorsi
- Extensor pollicis brevis
- Sartorius
- Extensor retinaculum
- Quadriceps femoris (vastus lateralis)
- Gluteus maximus
- Iliotibial tract
- Tibialis anterior
- Extensor digitorum longus
- Lateral head of gastrocnemius
- Fibularis (peroneus) longus
- Soleus
- Superior extensor retinaculum
- Inferior extensor retinaculum
- Tendo calcaneus (Achilles tendon)
- Superior peroneal retinaculum

Muscles of the Abdomen and Back

Muscles of the Abdomen—
Anterior View

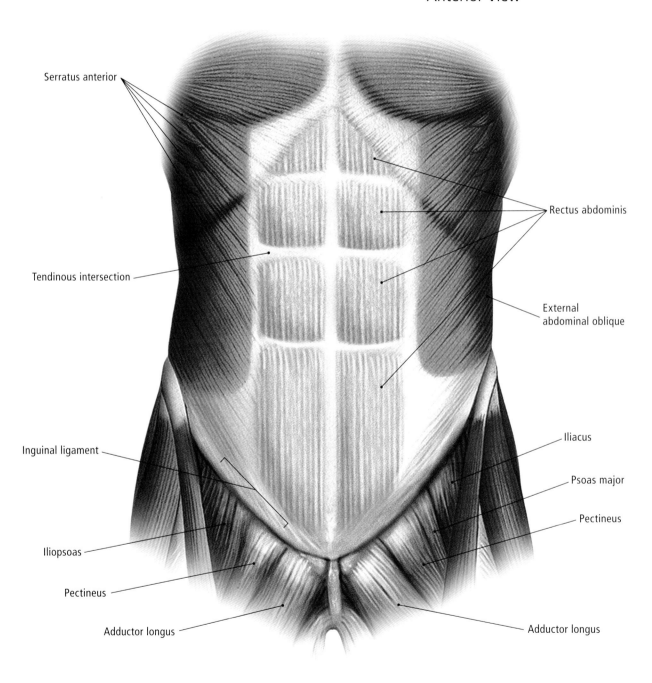

Serratus anterior

Tendinous intersection

Inguinal ligament

Iliopsoas

Pectineus

Adductor longus

Rectus abdominis

External
abdominal oblique

Iliacus

Psoas major

Pectineus

Adductor longus

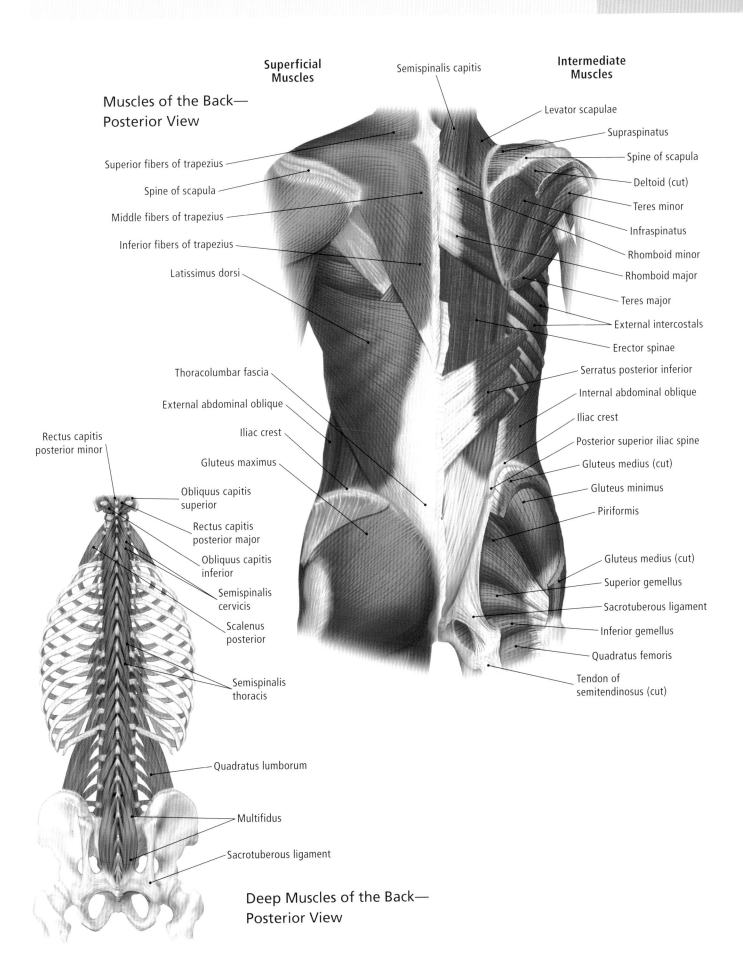

Superficial Muscles

Semispinalis capitis

Intermediate Muscles

Muscles of the Back— Posterior View

Levator scapulae

Supraspinatus

Superior fibers of trapezius

Spine of scapula

Spine of scapula

Deltoid (cut)

Middle fibers of trapezius

Teres minor

Infraspinatus

Inferior fibers of trapezius

Rhomboid minor

Rhomboid major

Latissimus dorsi

Teres major

External intercostals

Erector spinae

Serratus posterior inferior

Thoracolumbar fascia

Internal abdominal oblique

External abdominal oblique

Iliac crest

Iliac crest

Posterior superior iliac spine

Gluteus maximus

Gluteus medius (cut)

Rectus capitis posterior minor

Gluteus minimus

Obliquus capitis superior

Piriformis

Rectus capitis posterior major

Gluteus medius (cut)

Obliquus capitis inferior

Superior gemellus

Semispinalis cervicis

Sacrotuberous ligament

Scalenus posterior

Inferior gemellus

Quadratus femoris

Tendon of semitendinosus (cut)

Semispinalis thoracis

Quadratus lumborum

Multifidus

Sacrotuberous ligament

Deep Muscles of the Back— Posterior View

Muscles of the Upper and Lower Limb

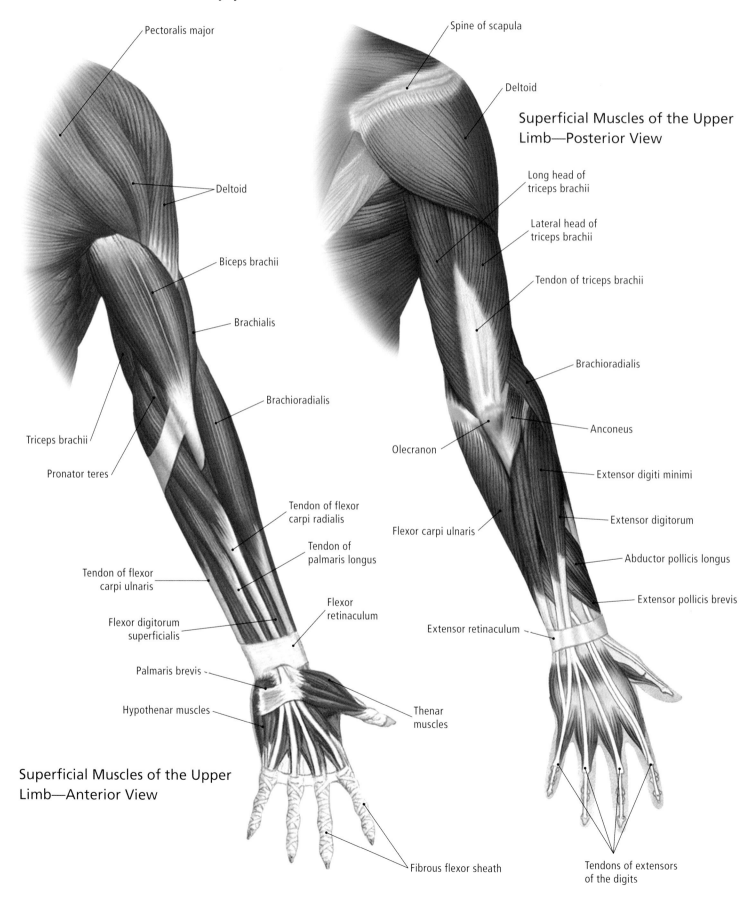

Pectoralis major

Spine of scapula

Deltoid

Superficial Muscles of the Upper Limb—Posterior View

Deltoid

Long head of triceps brachii

Biceps brachii

Lateral head of triceps brachii

Brachialis

Tendon of triceps brachii

Brachioradialis

Brachioradialis

Anconeus

Triceps brachii

Olecranon

Pronator teres

Extensor digiti minimi

Tendon of flexor carpi radialis

Flexor carpi ulnaris

Extensor digitorum

Tendon of palmaris longus

Abductor pollicis longus

Tendon of flexor carpi ulnaris

Extensor pollicis brevis

Flexor digitorum superficialis

Flexor retinaculum

Extensor retinaculum

Palmaris brevis

Hypothenar muscles

Thenar muscles

Superficial Muscles of the Upper Limb—Anterior View

Fibrous flexor sheath

Tendons of extensors of the digits

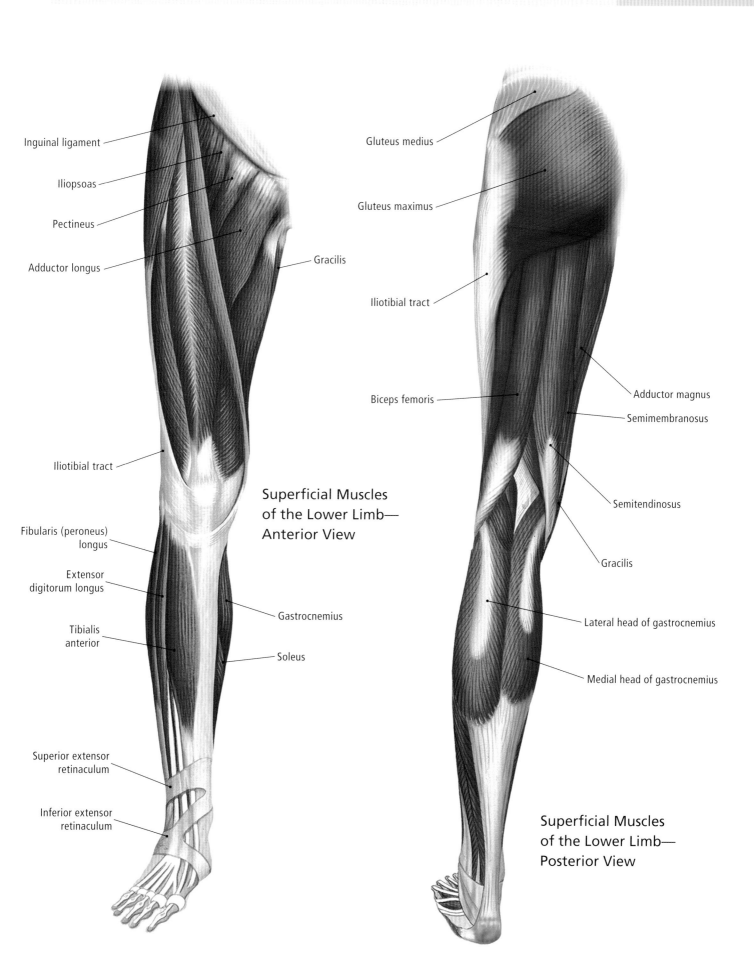

Inguinal ligament

Iliopsoas

Pectineus

Adductor longus

Gracilis

Iliotibial tract

Fibularis (peroneus) longus

Extensor digitorum longus

Tibialis anterior

Superior extensor retinaculum

Inferior extensor retinaculum

Gastrocnemius

Soleus

Superficial Muscles of the Lower Limb— Anterior View

Gluteus medius

Gluteus maximus

Iliotibial tract

Biceps femoris

Adductor magnus

Semimembranosus

Semitendinosus

Gracilis

Lateral head of gastrocnemius

Medial head of gastrocnemius

Superficial Muscles of the Lower Limb— Posterior View

Bones of the Body

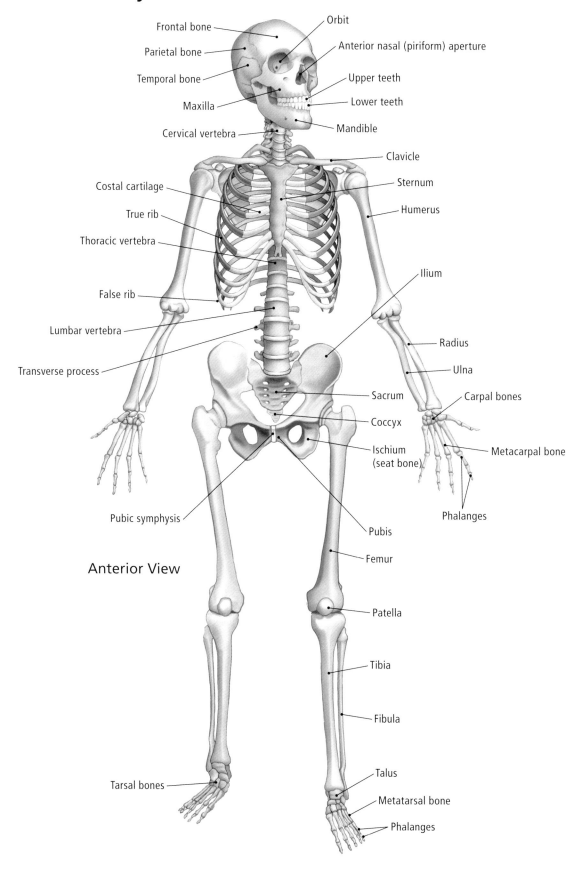

Frontal bone

Orbit

Parietal bone

Anterior nasal (piriform) aperture

Temporal bone

Upper teeth

Maxilla

Lower teeth

Cervical vertebra

Mandible

Clavicle

Costal cartilage

Sternum

True rib

Humerus

Thoracic vertebra

Ilium

False rib

Lumbar vertebra

Radius

Transverse process

Ulna

Sacrum

Carpal bones

Coccyx

Metacarpal bone

Ischium
(seat bone)

Phalanges

Pubic symphysis

Pubis

Anterior View

Femur

Patella

Tibia

Fibula

Talus

Tarsal bones

Metatarsal bone

Phalanges

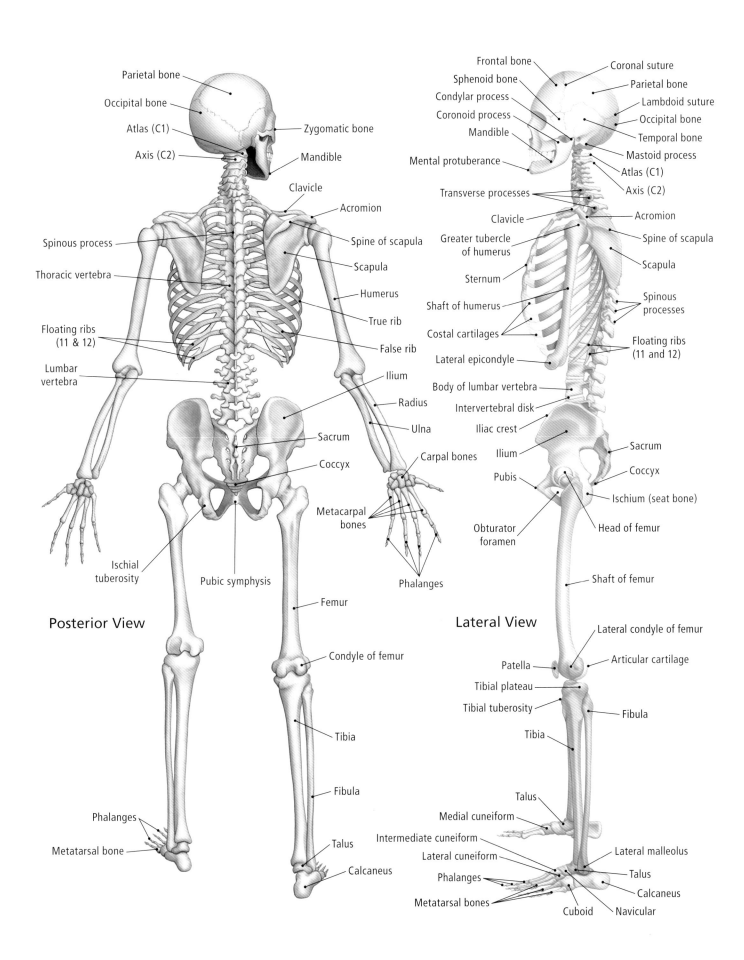

Posterior View

Lateral View

Parietal bone
Occipital bone
Atlas (C1)
Axis (C2)
Zygomatic bone
Mandible
Clavicle
Acromion
Spine of scapula
Spinous process
Scapula
Thoracic vertebra
Humerus
True rib
Floating ribs (11 & 12)
False rib
Lumbar vertebra
Ilium
Radius
Ulna
Sacrum
Coccyx
Carpal bones
Metacarpal bones
Ischial tuberosity
Pubic symphysis
Phalanges
Femur
Condyle of femur
Tibia
Fibula
Phalanges
Metatarsal bone
Talus
Calcaneus

Frontal bone
Coronal suture
Sphenoid bone
Parietal bone
Condylar process
Lambdoid suture
Coronoid process
Occipital bone
Mandible
Temporal bone
Mental protuberance
Mastoid process
Atlas (C1)
Axis (C2)
Transverse processes
Acromion
Clavicle
Spine of scapula
Greater tubercle of humerus
Scapula
Sternum
Spinous processes
Shaft of humerus
Floating ribs (11 and 12)
Costal cartilages
Lateral epicondyle
Body of lumbar vertebra
Intervertebral disk
Iliac crest
Sacrum
Ilium
Coccyx
Pubis
Ischium (seat bone)
Obturator foramen
Head of femur
Shaft of femur
Lateral condyle of femur
Articular cartilage
Patella
Tibial plateau
Tibial tuberosity
Fibula
Tibia
Talus
Medial cuneiform
Intermediate cuneiform
Lateral malleolus
Lateral cuneiform
Talus
Phalanges
Calcaneus
Metatarsal bones
Navicular
Cuboid

Vertebral Column

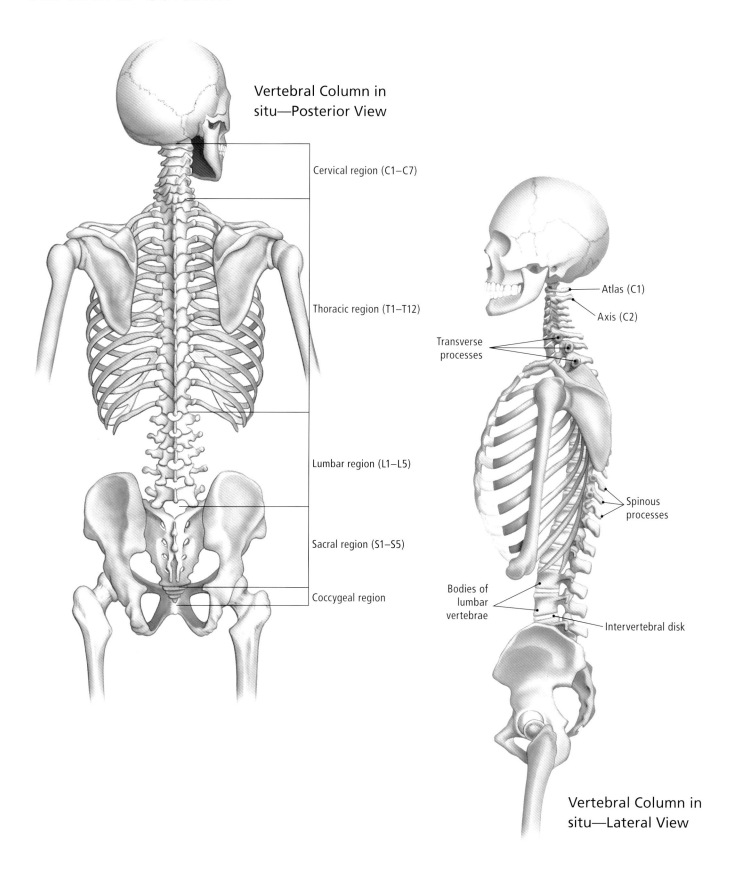

Vertebral Column in situ—Posterior View

Cervical region (C1–C7)

Thoracic region (T1–T12)

Lumbar region (L1–L5)

Sacral region (S1–S5)

Coccygeal region

Atlas (C1)

Axis (C2)

Transverse processes

Spinous processes

Bodies of lumbar vertebrae

Intervertebral disk

Vertebral Column in situ—Lateral View

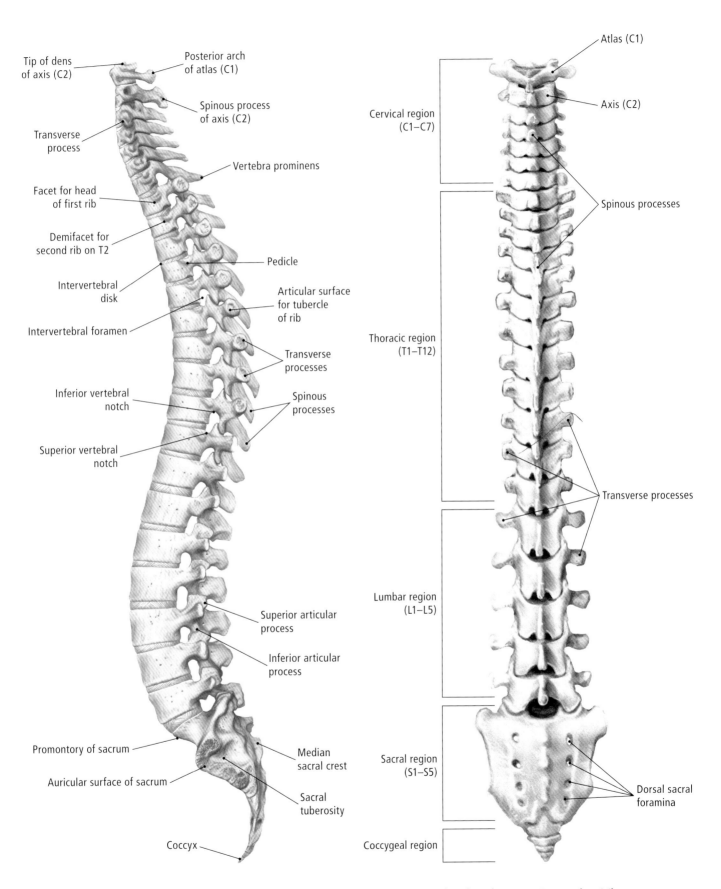

Tip of dens
of axis (C2)

Posterior arch
of atlas (C1)

Spinous process
of axis (C2)

Transverse
process

Vertebra prominens

Facet for head
of first rib

Demifacet for
second rib on T2

Intervertebral
disk

Pedicle

Intervertebral foramen

Articular surface
for tubercle
of rib

Transverse
processes

Inferior vertebral
notch

Spinous
processes

Superior vertebral
notch

Superior articular
process

Inferior articular
process

Promontory of sacrum

Auricular surface of sacrum

Median
sacral crest

Sacral
tuberosity

Coccyx

Atlas (C1)

Axis (C2)

Cervical region
(C1–C7)

Spinous processes

Thoracic region
(T1–T12)

Transverse processes

Lumbar region
(L1–L5)

Sacral region
(S1–S5)

Dorsal sacral
foramina

Coccygeal region

Vertebral Column—Lateral View

Vertebral Column—Posterior View

Bones of the Upper and Lower Limb

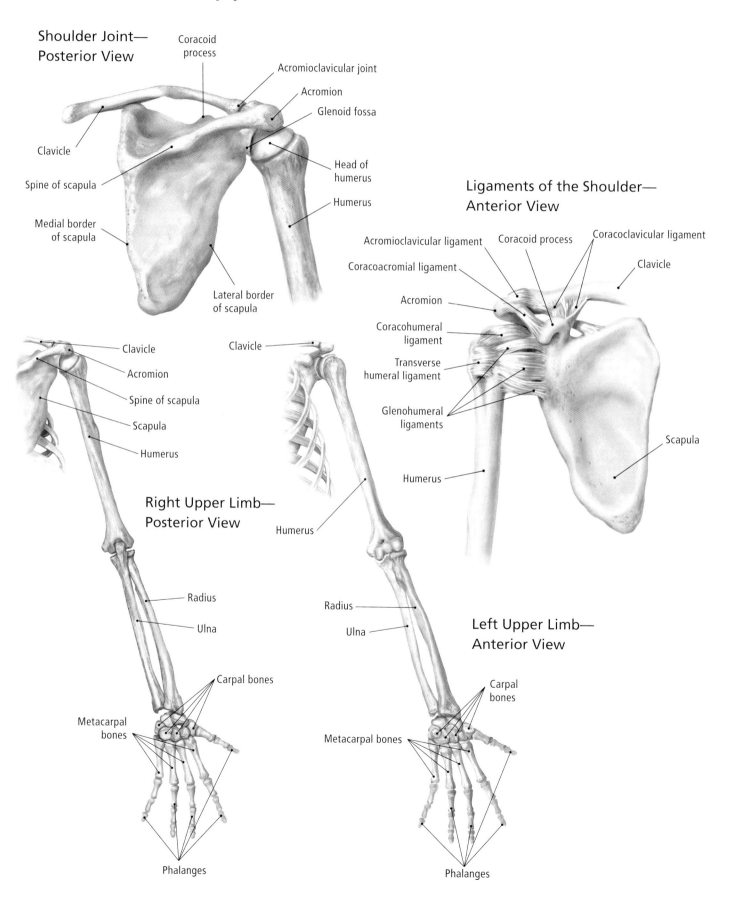

Shoulder Joint—
Posterior View

Coracoid process

Acromioclavicular joint

Acromion

Glenoid fossa

Clavicle

Head of humerus

Spine of scapula

Humerus

Medial border of scapula

Lateral border of scapula

Ligaments of the Shoulder—
Anterior View

Acromioclavicular ligament

Coracoid process

Coracoclavicular ligament

Coracoacromial ligament

Clavicle

Acromion

Coracohumeral ligament

Transverse humeral ligament

Glenohumeral ligaments

Scapula

Humerus

Clavicle

Acromion

Spine of scapula

Scapula

Humerus

Clavicle

Right Upper Limb—
Posterior View

Humerus

Radius

Ulna

Radius

Ulna

Left Upper Limb—
Anterior View

Carpal bones

Carpal bones

Metacarpal bones

Metacarpal bones

Phalanges

Phalanges

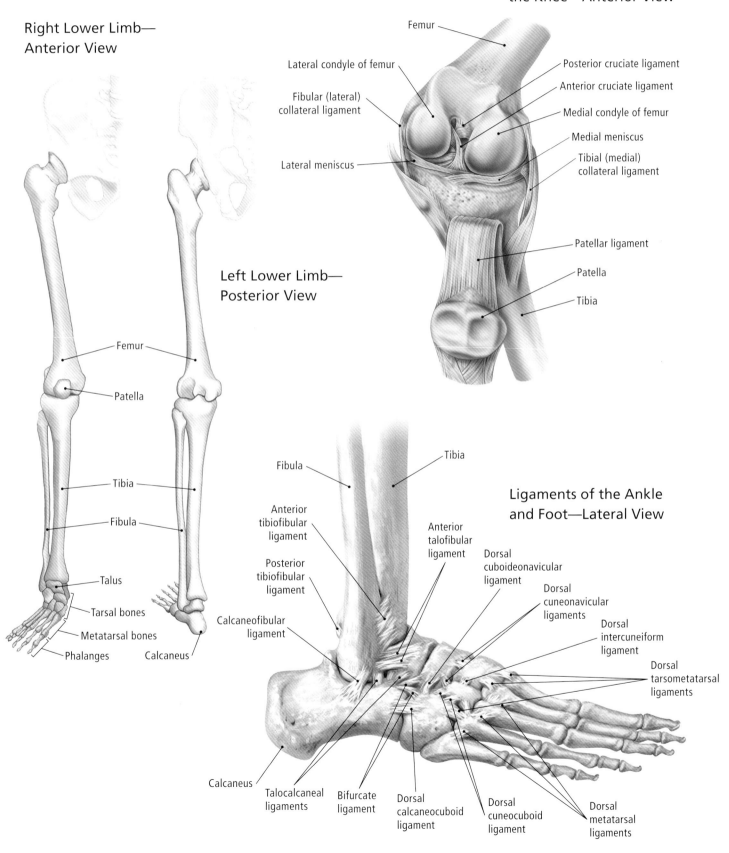

**Right Lower Limb—
Anterior View**

**Bones and Ligaments of
the Knee—Anterior View**

Femur

Lateral condyle of femur

Fibular (lateral)
collateral ligament

Posterior cruciate ligament

Anterior cruciate ligament

Medial condyle of femur

Medial meniscus

Tibial (medial)
collateral ligament

Lateral meniscus

Patellar ligament

Patella

Tibia

**Left Lower Limb—
Posterior View**

Femur

Patella

Tibia

Fibula

Talus

Tarsal bones

Metatarsal bones

Phalanges

Calcaneus

Fibula

Tibia

**Ligaments of the Ankle
and Foot—Lateral View**

Anterior
tibiofibular
ligament

Anterior
talofibular
ligament

Dorsal
cuboideonavicular
ligament

Dorsal
cuneonavicular
ligaments

Posterior
tibiofibular
ligament

Calcaneofibular
ligament

Dorsal
intercuneiform
ligament

Dorsal
tarsometatarsal
ligaments

Calcaneus

Talocalcaneal
ligaments

Bifurcate
ligament

Dorsal
calcaneocuboid
ligament

Dorsal
cuneocuboid
ligament

Dorsal
metatarsal
ligaments

Nervous System

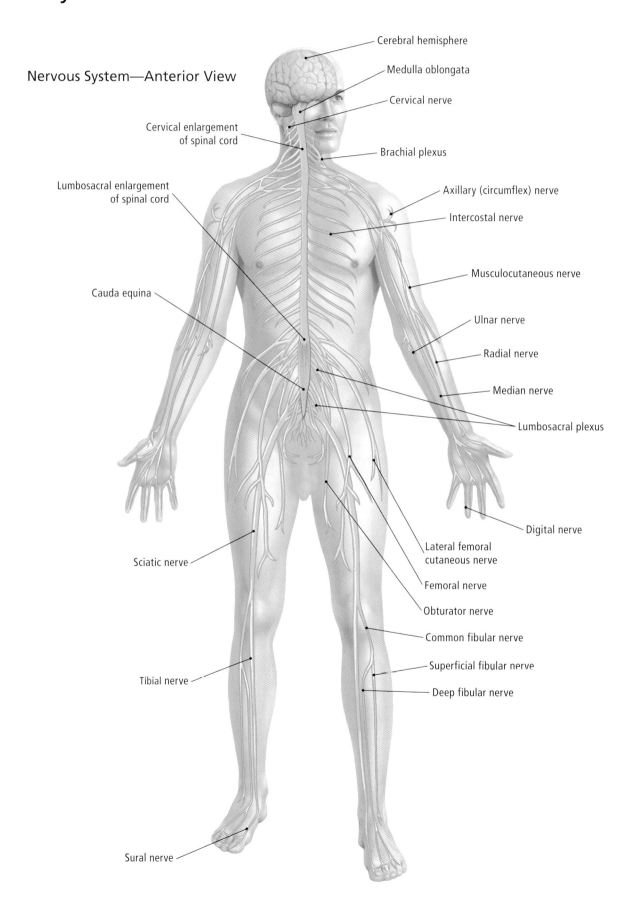

Nervous System—Anterior View

Cerebral hemisphere

Medulla oblongata

Cervical nerve

Cervical enlargement
of spinal cord

Brachial plexus

Lumbosacral enlargement
of spinal cord

Axillary (circumflex) nerve

Intercostal nerve

Musculocutaneous nerve

Ulnar nerve

Cauda equina

Radial nerve

Median nerve

Lumbosacral plexus

Digital nerve

Lateral femoral
cutaneous nerve

Sciatic nerve

Femoral nerve

Obturator nerve

Common fibular nerve

Superficial fibular nerve

Tibial nerve

Deep fibular nerve

Sural nerve

Central Nervous System

Autonomic Nervous System

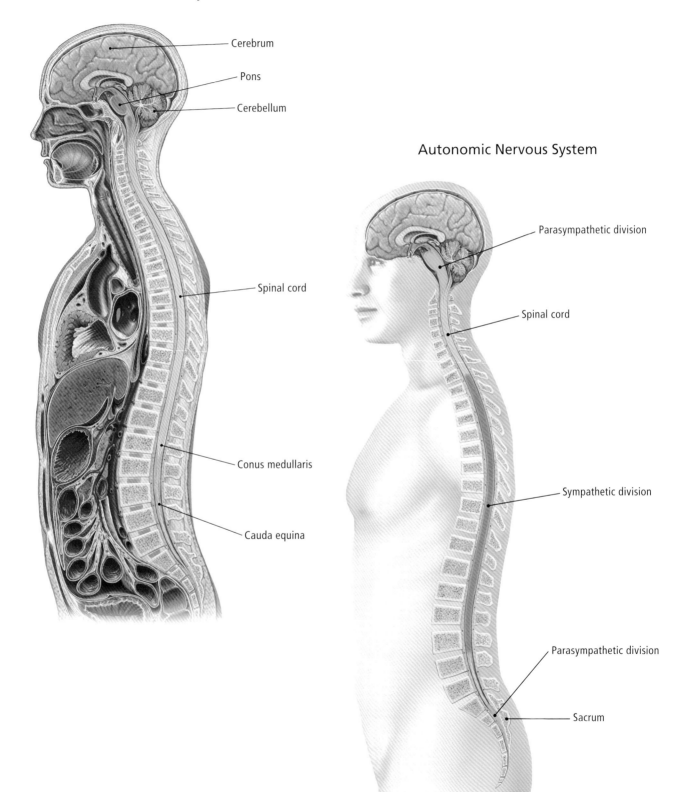

Cerebrum

Pons

Cerebellum

Spinal cord

Conus medullaris

Cauda equina

Parasympathetic division

Spinal cord

Sympathetic division

Parasympathetic division

Sacrum

Spinal Cord

Spinal Cord—Cross-Sectional View

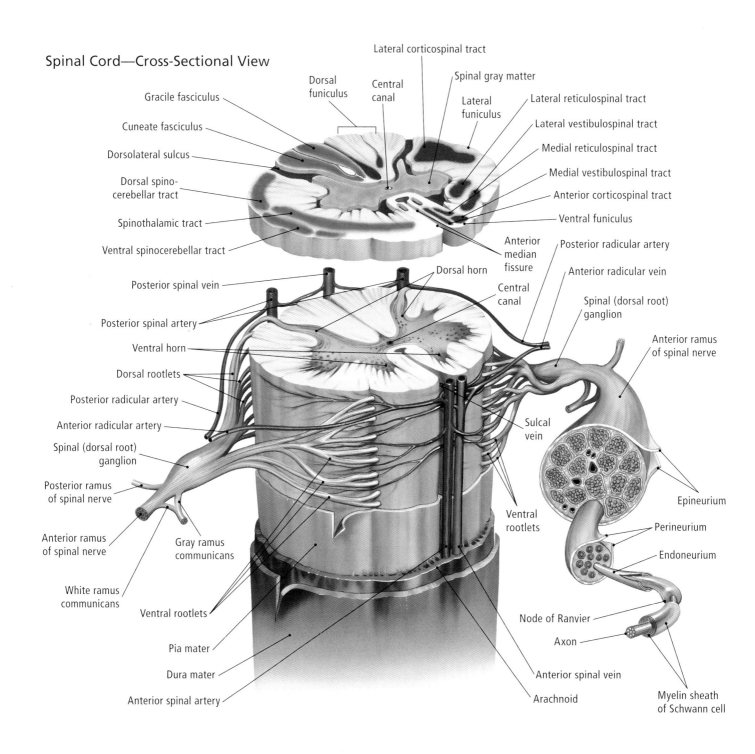

Lateral corticospinal tract
Dorsal funiculus
Central canal
Spinal gray matter
Gracile fasciculus
Lateral funiculus
Lateral reticulospinal tract
Cuneate fasciculus
Lateral vestibulospinal tract
Dorsolateral sulcus
Medial reticulospinal tract
Dorsal spino-cerebellar tract
Medial vestibulospinal tract
Spinothalamic tract
Anterior corticospinal tract
Ventral spinocerebellar tract
Ventral funiculus
Anterior median fissure
Posterior radicular artery
Posterior spinal vein
Dorsal horn
Anterior radicular vein
Central canal
Spinal (dorsal root) ganglion
Posterior spinal artery
Anterior ramus of spinal nerve
Ventral horn
Dorsal rootlets
Posterior radicular artery
Anterior radicular artery
Sulcal vein
Spinal (dorsal root) ganglion
Posterior ramus of spinal nerve
Epineurium
Anterior ramus of spinal nerve
Gray ramus communicans
Perineurium
White ramus communicans
Endoneurium
Ventral rootlets
Pia mater
Ventral rootlets
Node of Ranvier
Dura mater
Axon
Anterior spinal vein
Anterior spinal artery
Arachnoid
Myelin sheath of Schwann cell

Spinal Nerves

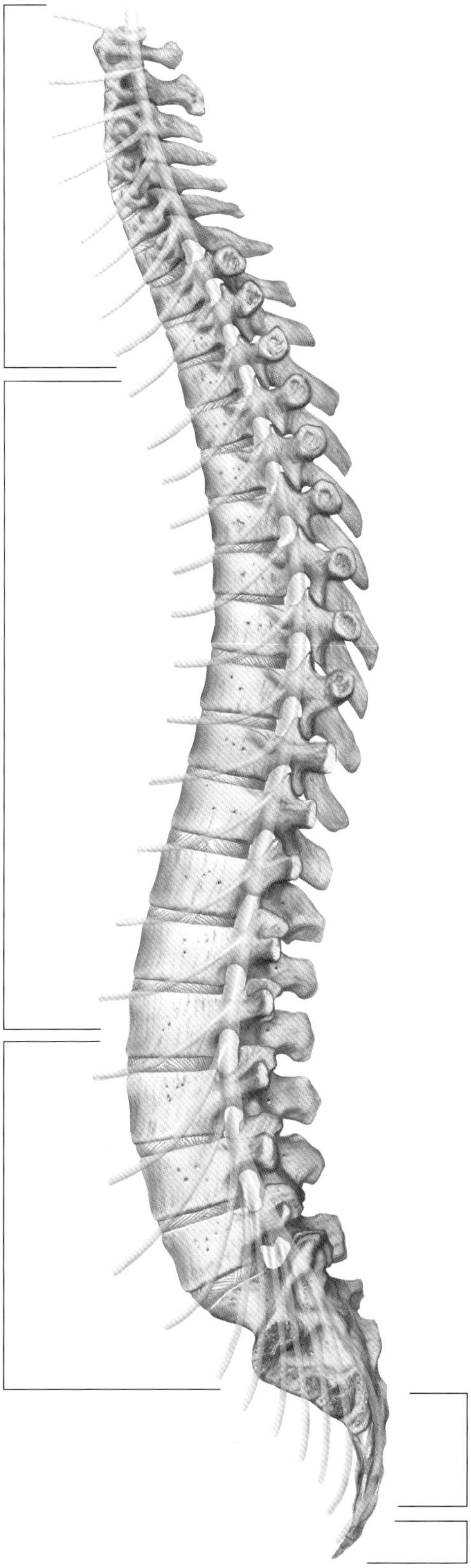

Spinal nerves C1–C8

Spinal nerves T1–T12

Spinal nerves L1–L5

Spinal nerves S1–S5

Coccygeal
spinal nerve

Spinal Cord—Anterior View

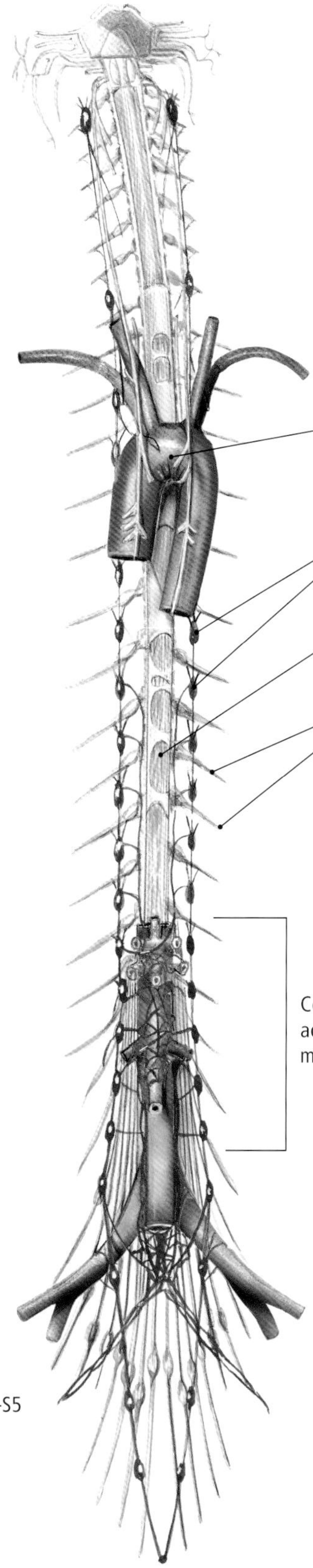

Aortic arch

Sympathetic ganglia

Spinal cord

Peripheral nerves

Celiac, superior mesenteric,
aorticorenal, and inferior
mesenteric plexuses

Circulatory System

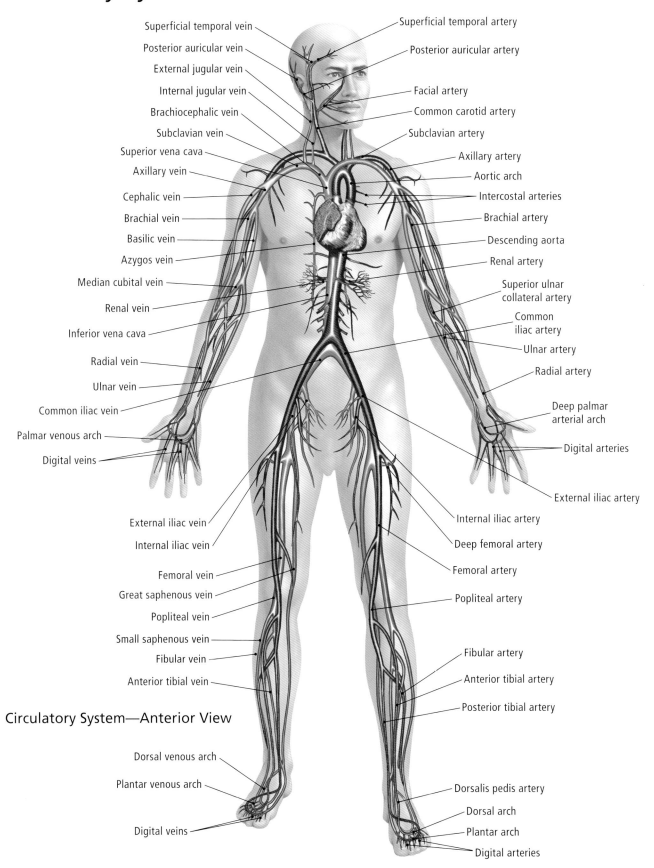

Superficial temporal vein

Posterior auricular vein

External jugular vein

Internal jugular vein

Brachiocephalic vein

Subclavian vein

Superior vena cava

Axillary vein

Cephalic vein

Brachial vein

Basilic vein

Azygos vein

Median cubital vein

Renal vein

Inferior vena cava

Radial vein

Ulnar vein

Common iliac vein

Palmar venous arch

Digital veins

Superficial temporal artery

Posterior auricular artery

Facial artery

Common carotid artery

Subclavian artery

Axillary artery

Aortic arch

Intercostal arteries

Brachial artery

Descending aorta

Renal artery

Superior ulnar collateral artery

Common iliac artery

Ulnar artery

Radial artery

Deep palmar arterial arch

Digital arteries

External iliac artery

Internal iliac artery

Deep femoral artery

Femoral artery

Popliteal artery

Fibular artery

Anterior tibial artery

Posterior tibial artery

External iliac vein

Internal iliac vein

Femoral vein

Great saphenous vein

Popliteal vein

Small saphenous vein

Fibular vein

Anterior tibial vein

Circulatory System—Anterior View

Dorsal venous arch

Plantar venous arch

Digital veins

Dorsalis pedis artery

Dorsal arch

Plantar arch

Digital arteries

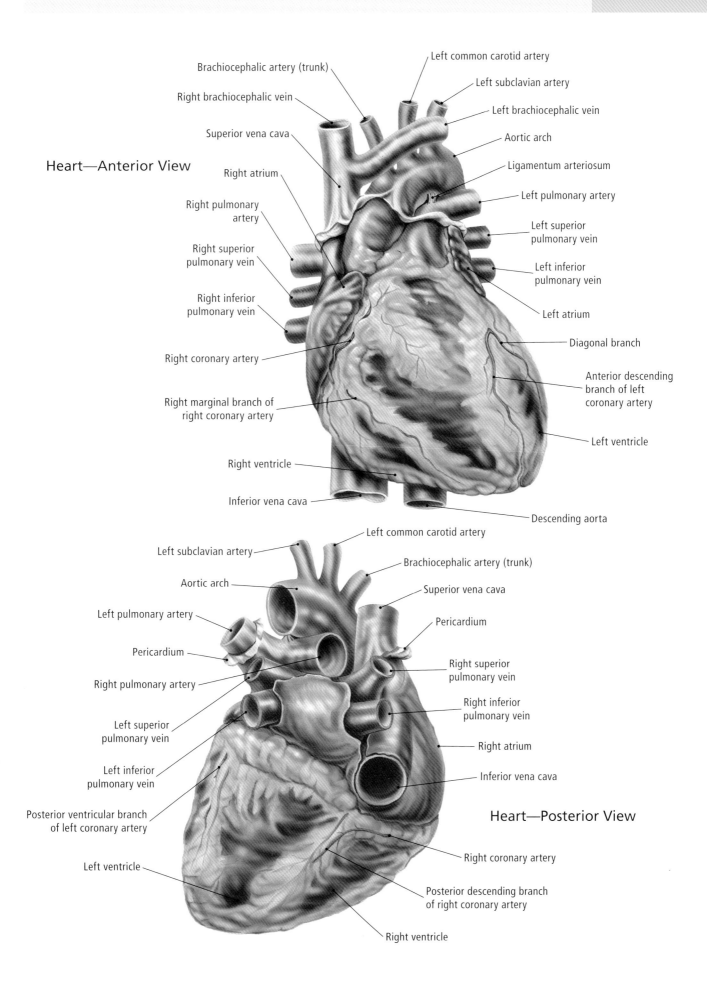

Heart—Anterior View

Brachiocephalic artery (trunk)
Right brachiocephalic vein
Superior vena cava
Right atrium
Right pulmonary artery
Right superior pulmonary vein
Right inferior pulmonary vein
Right coronary artery
Right marginal branch of right coronary artery
Right ventricle
Inferior vena cava

Left common carotid artery
Left subclavian artery
Left brachiocephalic vein
Aortic arch
Ligamentum arteriosum
Left pulmonary artery
Left superior pulmonary vein
Left inferior pulmonary vein
Left atrium
Diagonal branch
Anterior descending branch of left coronary artery
Left ventricle
Descending aorta

Left common carotid artery
Left subclavian artery
Brachiocephalic artery (trunk)
Aortic arch
Superior vena cava
Left pulmonary artery
Pericardium
Pericardium
Right superior pulmonary vein
Right pulmonary artery
Right inferior pulmonary vein
Left superior pulmonary vein
Right atrium
Left inferior pulmonary vein
Inferior vena cava
Posterior ventricular branch of left coronary artery
Left ventricle
Right coronary artery
Posterior descending branch of right coronary artery
Right ventricle

Heart—Posterior View

Blood Vessels of the Upper and Lower Limb

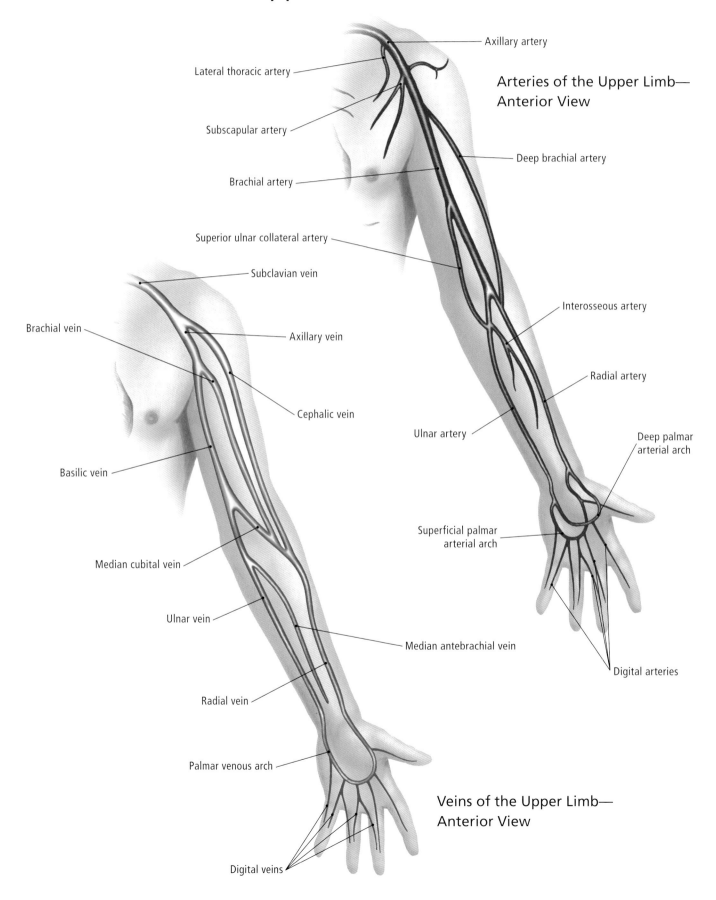

Lateral thoracic artery

Subscapular artery

Brachial artery

Superior ulnar collateral artery

Subclavian vein

Brachial vein

Axillary vein

Cephalic vein

Basilic vein

Median cubital vein

Ulnar vein

Median antebrachial vein

Radial vein

Palmar venous arch

Digital veins

Axillary artery

**Arteries of the Upper Limb—
Anterior View**

Deep brachial artery

Interosseous artery

Radial artery

Ulnar artery

Deep palmar
arterial arch

Superficial palmar
arterial arch

Digital arteries

**Veins of the Upper Limb—
Anterior View**

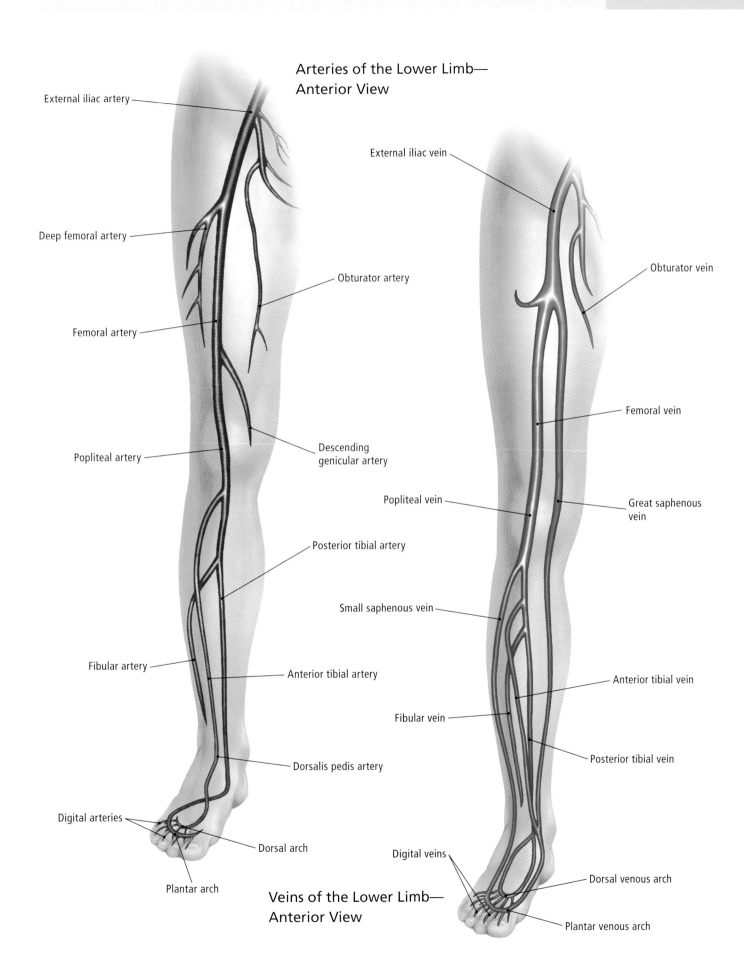

Arteries of the Lower Limb—
Anterior View

External iliac artery

Deep femoral artery

Femoral artery

Popliteal artery

Obturator artery

Descending
genicular artery

Posterior tibial artery

Fibular artery

Anterior tibial artery

Dorsalis pedis artery

Digital arteries

Dorsal arch

Plantar arch

External iliac vein

Obturator vein

Femoral vein

Popliteal vein

Great saphenous
vein

Small saphenous vein

Anterior tibial vein

Fibular vein

Posterior tibial vein

Digital veins

Dorsal venous arch

Plantar venous arch

Veins of the Lower Limb—
Anterior View

Respiratory System

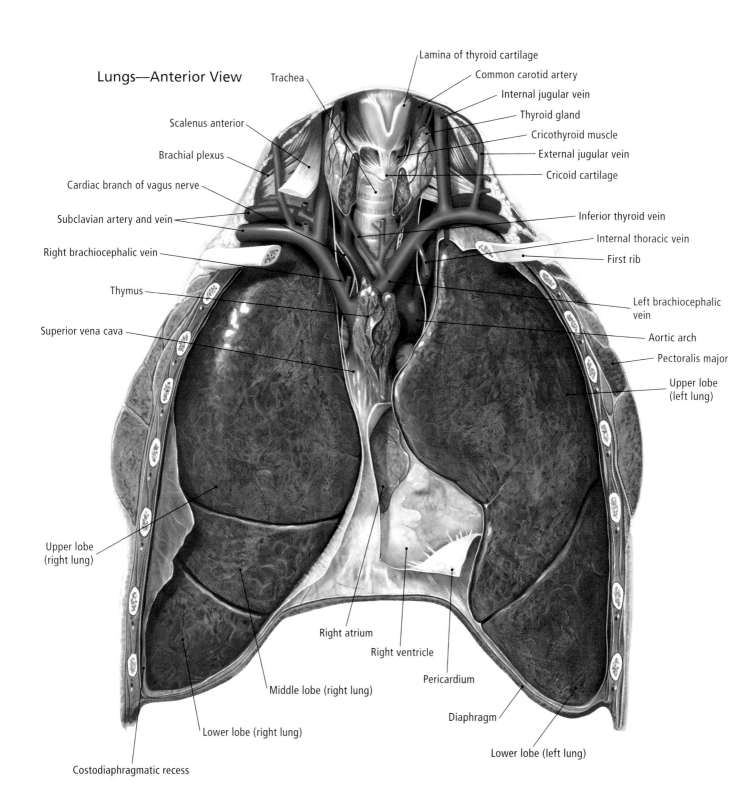

Lungs—Anterior View

- Lamina of thyroid cartilage
- Trachea
- Common carotid artery
- Internal jugular vein
- Thyroid gland
- Scalenus anterior
- Cricothyroid muscle
- Brachial plexus
- External jugular vein
- Cricoid cartilage
- Cardiac branch of vagus nerve
- Subclavian artery and vein
- Inferior thyroid vein
- Internal thoracic vein
- Right brachiocephalic vein
- First rib
- Thymus
- Left brachiocephalic vein
- Superior vena cava
- Aortic arch
- Pectoralis major
- Upper lobe (left lung)
- Upper lobe (right lung)
- Right atrium
- Right ventricle
- Pericardium
- Middle lobe (right lung)
- Diaphragm
- Lower lobe (right lung)
- Lower lobe (left lung)
- Costodiaphragmatic recess

Respiratory System—Anterior View

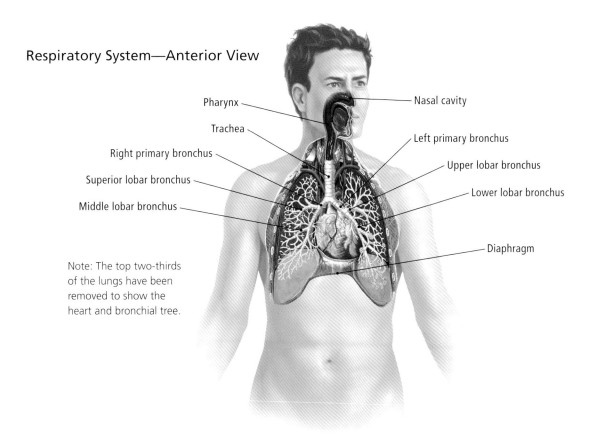

Pharynx

Nasal cavity

Trachea

Left primary bronchus

Right primary bronchus

Upper lobar bronchus

Superior lobar bronchus

Lower lobar bronchus

Middle lobar bronchus

Diaphragm

Note: The top two-thirds of the lungs have been removed to show the heart and bronchial tree.

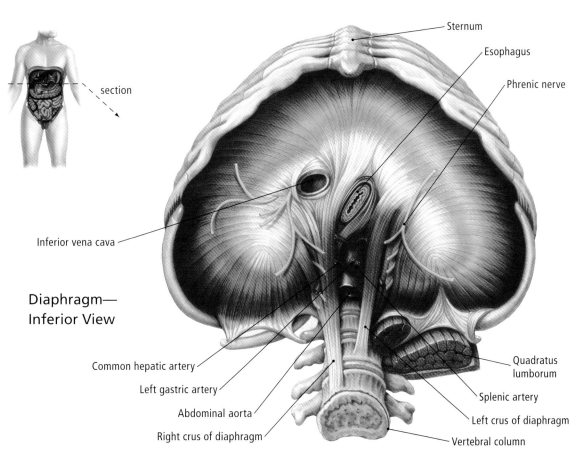

section

Diaphragm— Inferior View

Sternum

Esophagus

Phrenic nerve

Inferior vena cava

Common hepatic artery

Left gastric artery

Abdominal aorta

Right crus of diaphragm

Quadratus lumborum

Splenic artery

Left crus of diaphragm

Vertebral column

Movements of the Body

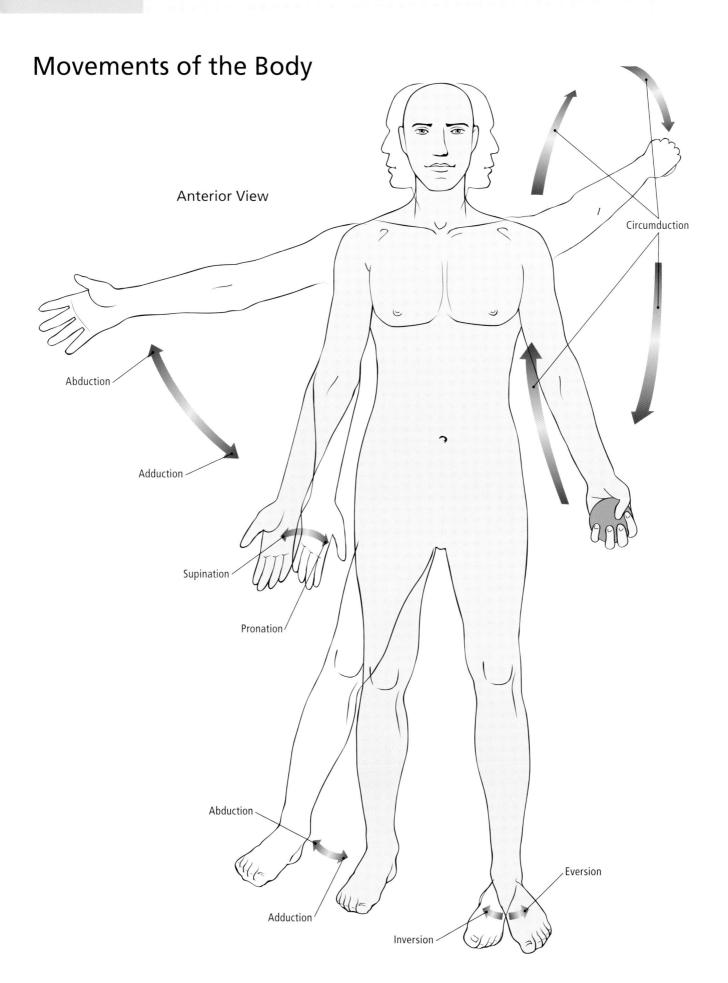

Anterior View

Circumduction

Abduction

Adduction

Supination

Pronation

Abduction

Adduction

Eversion

Inversion

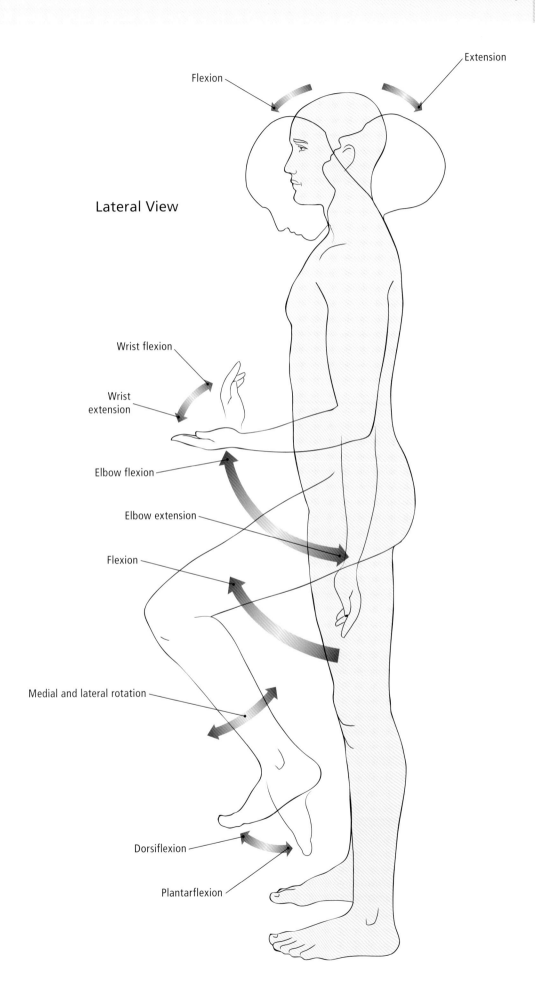

Lateral View

Flexion

Extension

Wrist flexion

Wrist extension

Elbow flexion

Elbow extension

Flexion

Medial and lateral rotation

Dorsiflexion

Plantarflexion

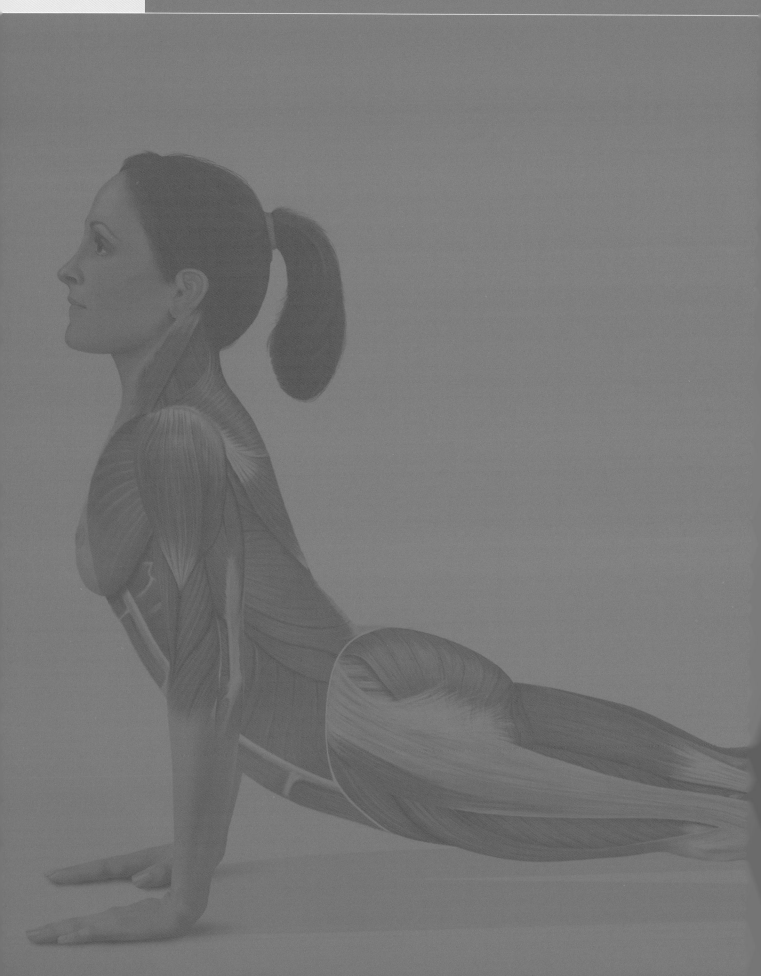

Principles of Yoga

Yoga is an approach to life that helps us on the path to
a more healthy and content way of being. It is an ancient
system that intertwines many physical and spiritual practices
that are designed not only to develop the body but also to
broaden our mental faculties and spiritual capacities. The
principles practiced within this system include focused
breathing, meditation, relaxation, and a healthy diet, and,
of course, exercise in the form of asanas, or postures, the
practice of which makes up the main content of this book.

What Is Yoga?

The word "yoga" comes from the Sanskrit word for "root," *yuj*, which in this context means "to join," "to yoke," or "to unite"—the union in this case is between the mind, body, and soul. This union is achieved through the physical and spiritual practices of yoga, which include yoga postures, meditation, and pranayama (yogic breathing exercises). When practicing yoga with complete devotion, this connection between the body and mind can ultimately lead to "samadhi," or bliss.

Yoga Philosophy— The Eight Limbs of Yoga

The practice of yoga does not just focus on physical postures to improve the body, but deals with all the aspects of our being. The "eight limbs of yoga" are steps in a person's journey toward harmony of the mind, body, and spirit.

They are:

1. **YAMA:** Our morals and ethical standards, and our behavior toward others.

2. **NIYAMA:** Our treatment of, and our attitude toward, ourselves.

3. **ASANA:** The regular practice of hatha yoga postures, through which we cultivate a healthy body and clear mind.

4. **PRANAYAMA:** A series of breath-control techniques that can lead to more efficient respiration; they highlight the connection between the breath, body, and mind.

5. **PRATYAHARA:** The practice of withdrawing the senses from the external world to turn focus inward, increasing the focus on the mind.

6. **DHARANA:** The art of concentration that, when practiced regularly, lets us focus completely, remaining uninterrupted by external or internal distractions.

7. **DHYANA:** Dharana (above) leads to dhyana, or meditation; a natural flow of energy between the self and the universe.

8. **SAMADHI:** The quiet state of blissful awareness, it is the culmination of the eight-limb path of yoga.

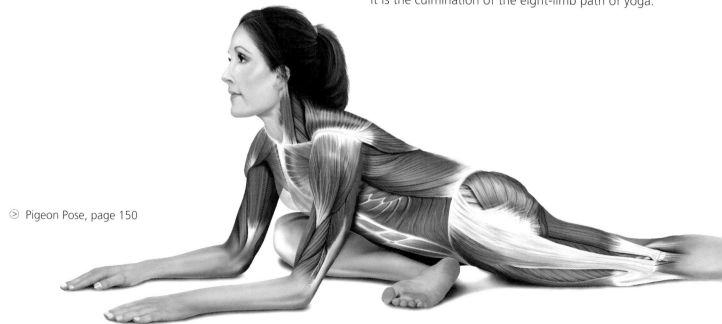

⊘ Pigeon Pose, page 150

The Chakras System

By working through the eight limbs of yoga, we can balance our "subtle body." The subtle body is something you can't see or touch—it's where your energy flows. Chakras are believed to be the energy centers in the subtle body, lying within the spinal cord and corresponding to the main nerve centers in the body. They can affect both the subtle and physical body, transforming subtle energy into physical energy and back again.

There are seven main chakras and it is believed that by balancing our chakra system, we can lead healthier and happier lives.

The seven chakras are:

1. MULADHARA: The root chakra; located at the bottom of the spine.

2. SVADHISTHANA: The sacral chakra; located at the ovaries or prostate.

3. MANIPURA: The solar plexus chakra; located in the navel area.

4. ANAHATA: The heart chakra; located at the heart area.

5. VISSUDHA: The throat chakra; located in the throat and neck area.

6. AJNA: The brow, or third eye, chakra; located at the pineal gland (in the brain).

7. SAHASRARA: The crown chakra; located at the crown of the head.

Each chakra is located along the spine, starting at the bottom and running up to the crown of the head. Each radiates a specific color and spiritual quality, and together they make up the psychological, physical, and emotional states necessary for the development of the whole person. The three chakras residing below the heart are mainly concerned with the physical body and physical needs; the chakras above the heart are of a more spiritual nature.

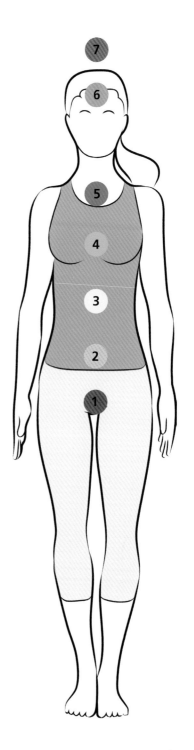

⊛ The seven chakras, and their position on the body.

Origins and History of Yoga

Until recently, many Western scholars thought that yoga originated around 500 BCE, during the time of Gautama the Buddha. However, the discovery of engravings in the ruins of two cities of the Indus civilization revealed that the origins reached back much farther, to at least 5,000 years ago. Yoga has developed continuously since its origins and can be divided into five major periods: vedic yoga, preclassical yoga, classical yoga, postclassical yoga, and modern yoga.

Vedic Yoga

This Sanskrit word "veda" means knowledge. *The Vedas*, the scriptures from this period, comprise a collection of texts, songs, mantras, and rituals meant for use by a Vedic priest. The ancient yoga text the Rig Veda contains teachings about the praise of higher power and forms the origins of today's Hindu religion.

Preclassical Yoga

This covers the period from about 2000 BCE to the second century CE, during which the Upanishads were created. These philosophical texts teach about the sacrifice of the ego through self-knowledge, action, and wisdom, and the hidden unity of all things. They also contain the first reference to yoga as a path through which the student can gain freedom from suffering and offer some instruction on how this can be achieved.

Classical Yoga

This relates to the period defined by Sage Patañjali's eight-limb yoga, as taught in his text *The Yoga Sutra*. *The Yoga Sutra* was the first systematic presentation of yoga and has been scrutinized, interpreted, and commented on throughout the centuries since it was written. Patañjali presented the "eight-limb path," which outlines the stages toward obtaining enlightenment. The text is thought to have been written during the second century CE, and it strongly influences many modern styles of yoga.

Postclassical Yoga

Postclassical yoga differs from the yoga of other eras in that its goal is no longer liberation of the person from their reality but instead that they accept their own reality and attempt to live in the moment. Its teachings refer to "vedanta," which represents a philosophical approach to the teachings of the Vedas, in particular, the Upanishads.

The yoga masters of this time created practices designed to rejuvenate and energize the body and prolong physical life. The ultimate aim of some of these practices was to energize the physical body to such a degree that the physical structure changed and the body became immortal. This is the origin of the modern yoga era, and of hatha yoga.

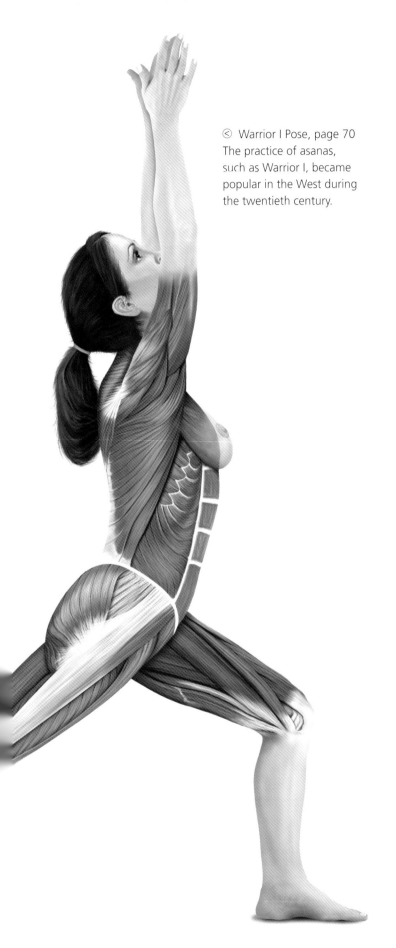

⊙ Warrior I Pose, page 70
The practice of asanas,
such as Warrior I, became
popular in the West during
the twentieth century.

Modern Yoga

This refers to the period in the nineteenth century during which numerous yoga masters brought their teachings to the United States and Europe. It was with the arrival of Swami Vivekananda, an Indian Hindu monk, in the United States, and his representation of India at the Parliament of World Religions in 1893, that the physical approach to yoga, known as hatha yoga, began to attract interest in the West.

Nearly thirty years later, in 1920, Paramahansa Yogananda arrived in Boston, Massachusetts, and established the Self-Realization Fellowship, which continues to have a wide following today. Other great modern teachers include Sri Krishnamacharya, who died at the age of 101 in 1989. His students included his son T. K. V. Desikachar, B. K. S. Iyengar, Indra Devi, and Sri K. Pattabhi Jois. All these students became teachers and were influential in spreading their knowledge of hatha yoga during the twentieth century. Their teachings are still practiced throughout the world today.

Hatha Yoga

Hatha yoga is the practice of asanaa (yoga postures). The word "hatha" comprises *ha* (meaning "sun") and *tha* (meaning "moon"), which refers to the balance of different aspects that are within all of us. This balance is achieved by regularly practicing sequences of asanas, which, as well as making the body strong and flexible, are intended to align the many energy channels of the body. In this way, hatha yoga is a path toward creating balance at all levels.

Many styles of hatha yoga are practiced today. Two of these, ashtanga yoga and Iyengar yoga, are especially popular in the West. These styles were popularized by Sri K. Pattabhi Jois and B. K. S. Iyengar respectively, and it is these two styles that form the basis of this book.

Yoga and Breathing

Breathing is one physical function that, although involuntary—meaning it occurs without instruction from our consciousness—can nevertheless be controlled. When we are not thinking about our breath, it continues to perform its vital functions of inhaling oxygen and exhaling carbon dioxide.

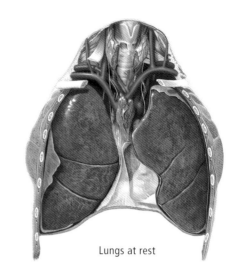

Lungs at rest

The nervous system is responsible for the regulation of breathing and controls the contractions of the muscles that make it happen. The process of breathing starts from a cluster of cells in the brain stem, collectively known as the respiratory center, that send impulses to the muscles involved; the key muscles used are the intercostals (between the ribs) and the diaphragm.

Pranayama

Pranayama is a yogic practice that increases our awareness of the physical processes involved in breathing, and in doing so allows for us to have more control over them.

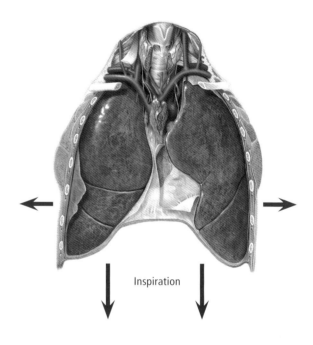

Inspiration

With regular practice of breath control, we can increase the amount of air we take into the lungs, leading to increased oxygenation of the blood. This is thought to help repair the body at a cellular level. Controlling the breath through pranayama is known to lower the heart rate and blood pressure, improving the efficiency of the body in utilizing oxygen. When the body works efficiently in this way, it has less physical stress placed upon it. This helps the mind to become calm and easier to control—which is one of the main aims of yoga.

During the practice of yoga asana, we should aim to lengthen both the inward breath and the outward breath, subtly energizing the body. Our breathing during yoga can also give an indication of whether we are working too strongly and putting undue strain on the body. If the breath is shallow and erratic, the body is being overexerted and will become tense. This is a sign that the yoga practice should be gentler so that the breath can again become slow and steady.

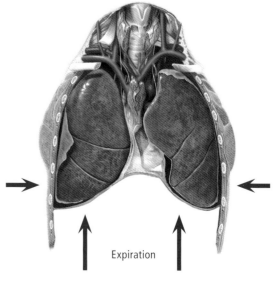

Expiration

Breath-Control Techniques

There are several pranayama techniques that can be used as part of a yoga practice. The two most common and accessible of these are outlined below:

Victorious Breath (*Ujjayi* Breathing)

This technique is energizing and relaxing, and the sound it produces is often likened to the sound of the ocean. Practice the breath by inhaling slightly more deeply than normal and, with the mouth closed, exhaling through the nose. The muscles of the throat will remain slightly constricted throughout, and this action of the throat creates a "Haaaa" sound. Ujjayi breathing can be performed in a sitting position and is especially effective when done during asana practice.

Alternate Nostril Breathing (*Nadi Shodhan*)

This is a simple breathing technique that works therapeutically to improve respiration and circulation. It also releases accumulated stress in the mind and body effectively.

Practice the breath by sitting comfortably with the spine straight and the left hand placed on the left knee, with the palm facing up. Tuck in the tips of the index finger and middle finger of the right hand toward the palm; if this is not possible, extend the fingers with the tips resting lightly on the "third eye" point, in between the eyebrows. Close the right nostril with the thumb, and inhale through the left nostril. Then close the left nostril with the second finger and little finger, remove the thumb, and exhale through the right nostril. Inhale through the right nostril. Now press the thumb on the right nostril again, lift the second and little finger from the left nostril, and release the breath gently through the left nostril. This is one cycle of alternate nostril breathing.

This technique is usually practiced for two minutes to begin with, gradually increasing to five minutes.

ⓢ **Breathing**

When we breathe in, the intercostal muscles move the ribs upward and outward and the diaphragm pushes downward. This draws air into the expanded lungs.

ⓥ During Shoulder Stand Pose (page 172) the "chin-lock" position of the neck, and the effect of gravity pushing down on the diaphragm, encourage deep abdominal breathing.

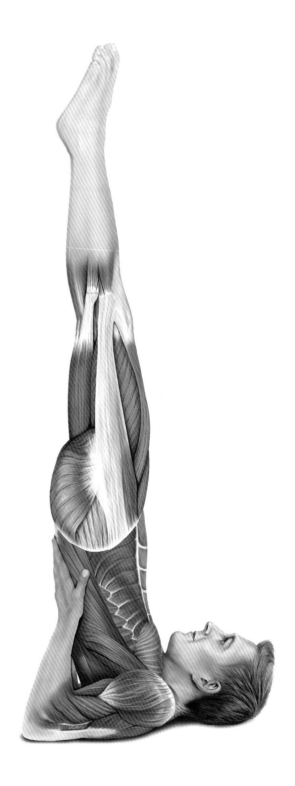

Yoga and the Spine

When viewed from the side, an adult spine has a natural S-shape curve. The neck and lower back regions have a slight concave curve, and the thoracic and sacral regions have a slight convex curve. The purpose of these curves is to absorb shock, maintain balance, and allow for range of motion throughout the spinal column.

For the spine to remain healthy, it is important that these natural curves of the spine are maintained. This can be achieved through the regular practice of a yoga program that stretches and strengthens the spinal column as an entire unit.

Yoga creates flexibility around the vertebrae and intervertebral disks and strengthens the supportive network of muscles, ligaments, and tendons. Space is created between the vertebrae, easing pressure on the disks, while circulation is improved, helping regeneration at a cellular level. Bone density is also increased, helping to minimize degeneration of the bones.

A balanced yoga program should include asanas that move the spine into and out of rotation, lateral flexion, forward flexion, and extension. When all these types of movements are practiced regularly, the spine will adopt a neutral alignment and negative postural patterns can be avoided. Good posture helps us to breathe more freely and improves our well-being by helping us to avoid muscle tightness and weakness that can contribute to backache.

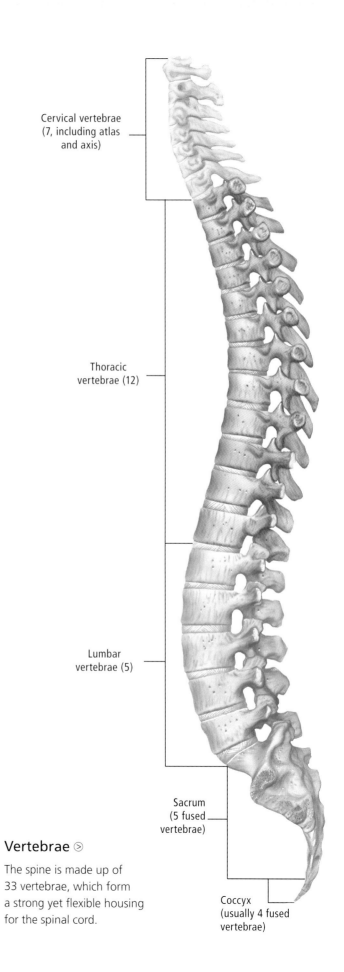

Cervical vertebrae
(7, including atlas
and axis)

Thoracic
vertebrae (12)

Lumbar
vertebrae (5)

Sacrum
(5 fused
vertebrae)

Coccyx
(usually 4 fused
vertebrae)

Vertebrae ⊚

The spine is made up of 33 vertebrae, which form a strong yet flexible housing for the spinal cord.

Joints and Movement

A well-balanced yoga program should incorporate as many different ranges of movement as possible to keep each joint functioning well. Within the skeleton there are three types of joints, which are categorized according to the degree of movement that each allows.

Types of Joints

The bones of **fibrous joints** are connected by fibrous tissue that allows for no movement (examples include where the bones of the skull join). The bones of **cartilaginous joints** are joined by cartilage. These joints must provide stability and so do not allow for a great deal of movement. Examples include the sacroiliac joint, where the spine meets the pelvis, and the sternocostal joints, where the front ribs attach to the sternum (breast bone).

The bones of **synovial joints** meet in a joint capsule. Examples include the knee joint, where the femur and tibia meet, and the elbow joint, where the humerus meets with the radius and ulna. These joints are the most common and most mobile joints, and it is these that we will mostly be referring to in this book. The body has six types of synovial joints, and their range of movement can be increased with regular hatha yoga practice.

ⓥ The three basic planes used to describe human anatomy.

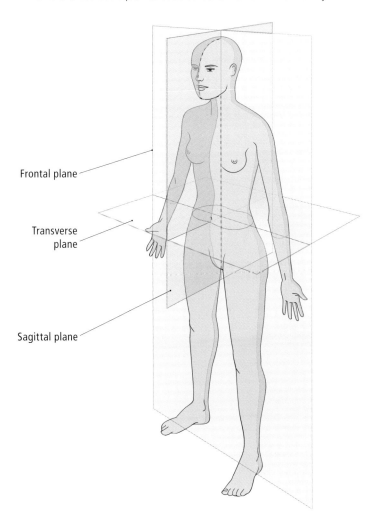

Frontal plane

Transverse plane

Sagittal plane

Planes of Movement

Movements of the body can be categorized into types by the direction in which they occur (see page 36). These types of movements also occur within a plane of movement. An anatomical plane is effectively an imaginary line—vertical or horizontal—drawn through the body.

There are three basic planes used in human anatomy:

The frontal plane is vertical and divides the body into back (posterior) and front (anterior) portions.

The transverse plane is parallel to the ground and separates the top half of the body from the lower half of the body.

The sagittal plane is vertical and divides the body into left and right portions.

These can be used to help describe movement. For example, by moving into Warrior I Pose (page 70), the front leg is in flexion at both the hip joint and knee joint while the back leg is extended. Both of these movements occur in the sagittal plane. The arms are abducted out to each side and up overhead in a frontal plane. If the upper body then moved on to Revolved Extended Side-Angle Pose (page 82), the spine and torso would then move on a transverse plane around a frontal axis point.

Types of Muscle Activity

The muscles of the body are divided into three main types: skeletal, smooth, and cardiac. Skeletal muscles are those attached to the skeleton, and it is these that produce movement by shortening and pulling on a bone via its tendon—it is these that we focus on in this book.

Most muscles work in opposing pairs to enable active extension and flexion in the joints. When one contracts and shortens, the other lengthens in response, and vice versa. When we stretch in hatha yoga, we are focusing mainly on muscles that lengthen as a result of another muscle shortening. For the purposes of hatha yoga, muscle contractions can be divided into two main types: isotonic and isometric.

Isotonic Muscle Contraction

When a muscle changes length to create movement, it is called an isotonic contraction. Isotonic muscle contractions can be divided into either concentric or eccentric activity.

Concentric activity is when the muscle shortens to create movement. An example of this is bending the knee joint from straight to flexed, as in Shoulder Bridge Pose

ⓥ Shoulder Bridge Pose, p.168
To achieve this bend at the knees, the hamstrings concentrically contract, acting as prime movers. The quadriceps must lengthen to allow this movement, acting as antagonists.

(page 168), which causes a concentric contraction of the hamstring muscles. When a muscle creates a concentric contraction, it is known as a **prime mover**, or **agonist**.

Eccentric muscle activity is when the muscle lengthens to allow for movement. In the example above, to let the knee bend, the opposing muscles—the quadriceps—need to lengthen via an eccentric muscle contraction. An eccentric muscle is also known as an **antagonist**.

To create stable, coordinated movement, other muscles often contract or provide assistance to the prime mover. These muscles are known as **synergists**. For example, if the knee joint bends, the gastrocnemius muscle (located at the back of the lower leg) contracts to assist the hamstring muscles with this movement; in this case, the gastrocnemius works as a synergist.

Isometric Muscle Contraction

Isometric contractions cause no change in the length of the muscle, but the muscle holds, or fixates, the body in position. For example, in Boat Pose (page 128), the rectus abdominis muscle group does not lengthen or shorten, but it contracts to hold the spine in place once the body has been moved into position. In this instance, the rectus abdominis muscle group would be known as a **fixator**.

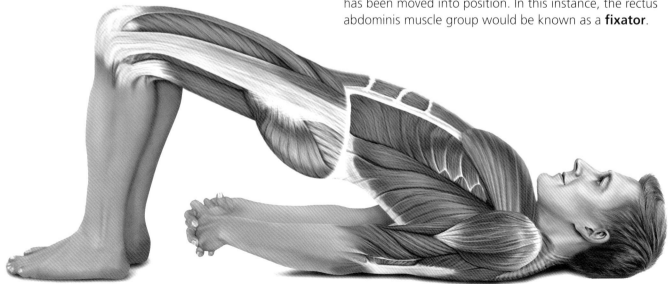

Types of Muscle Activity

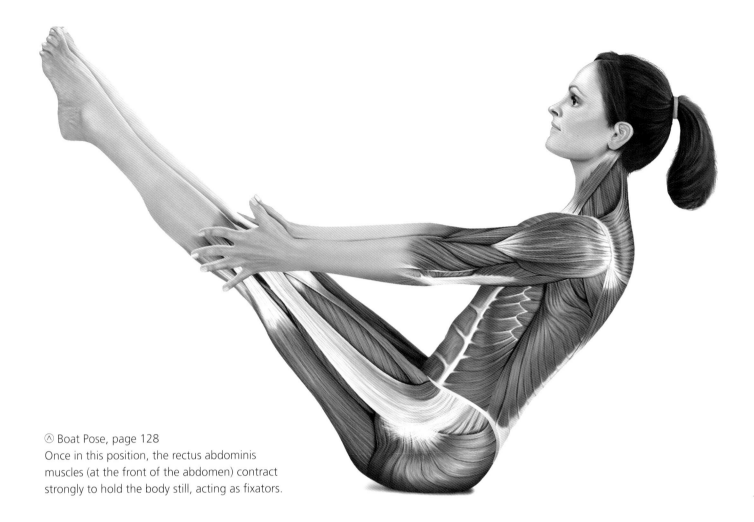

⊗ Boat Pose, page 128
Once in this position, the rectus abdominis
muscles (at the front of the abdomen) contract
strongly to hold the body still, acting as fixators.

In summary:

- **Prime movers** produce the initial movement of a joint.
  These are also known as **agonists** and produce
  movement via a concentric contraction.

- **Antagonists** lengthen to allow for the shortening
  of the prime mover, or agonist. This is an eccentric
  contraction.

- **Concentric muscle activity**—the muscle shortens to
  create movement.

- **Eccentric muscle activity**—the muscle lengthens to
  allow for movement. Also called **antagonists**.

- **Synergists** contract to assist the prime mover.

- **Fixators** contract statically to stabilize the position
  adopted, once the movement has occurred.

For the purposes of the muscle activity examined in this
book, the main muscle activity has been divided into
prime movers—those that initiate the movement by
shortening; and **antagonists**—those that allow for the
movement by lengthening.

Levers and Intensity

The lever system is well established in physics, and it is an important factor in yoga—without levers, movement could not occur, and they determine the intensity of each movement.

What Is a Lever?

All levers are made up of three elements:

- An axis point, also known as a fulcrum
- A load, also known as resistance or weight
- An effort, also known as the force

Collectively, the bones, ligaments, tendons, and muscles of the human body form levers to create movement. A joint forms the axis point and the muscles crossing the joint apply the effort, which then moves the lever, which, in turn, moves the load.

If we change the load or move the axis point, we change the effort the muscle has to exert to move the load. This means we can change the level of intensity levers experience, and so make particular movements of the body harder to achieve and maintain. An example of this outside of human anatomy is a children's seesaw. This has its axis point in the middle of the board and, because of this, the board will have an even load placed upon it (gravity) at each end. This means the board will remain parallel to the ground. If, however, we move the axis point to the left, for example, making the right side of the board longer, we have increased the load (gravity) at this end. The right side of the board will sink lower to the ground. This is a simple example of how moving the positioning of the axis changes the action of the lever.

Types of Levers

There are three different types of lever in the human body: first-class levers, second-class levers, and third-class levers.

First-class lever

A first-class lever has its axis located between the load and the effort. There are not many first-class levers in the human body; however, one example is the joint between the head and the first vertebra of the neck. The load is the head, the axis is the joint, and the muscular action (effort) comes from the posterior muscles attached to the skull, such as the trapezius. Therefore, if the upper trapezius muscles contract and shorten, they will be working against the weight of the head and gravity, and the chin will lift away from the chest and tilt backward. An example of this can be found in Upward-Facing Dog (page 146), where the chin is lifted a little.

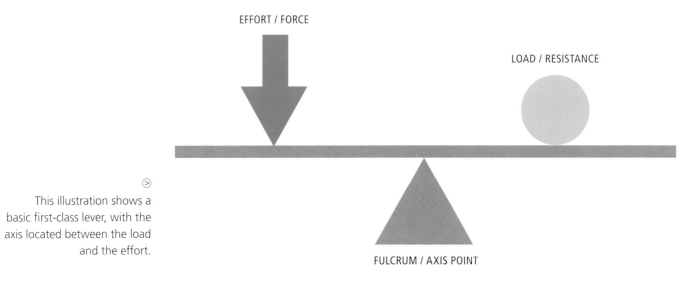

EFFORT / FORCE

LOAD / RESISTANCE

FULCRUM / AXIS POINT

⊛
This illustration shows a basic first-class lever, with the axis located between the load and the effort.

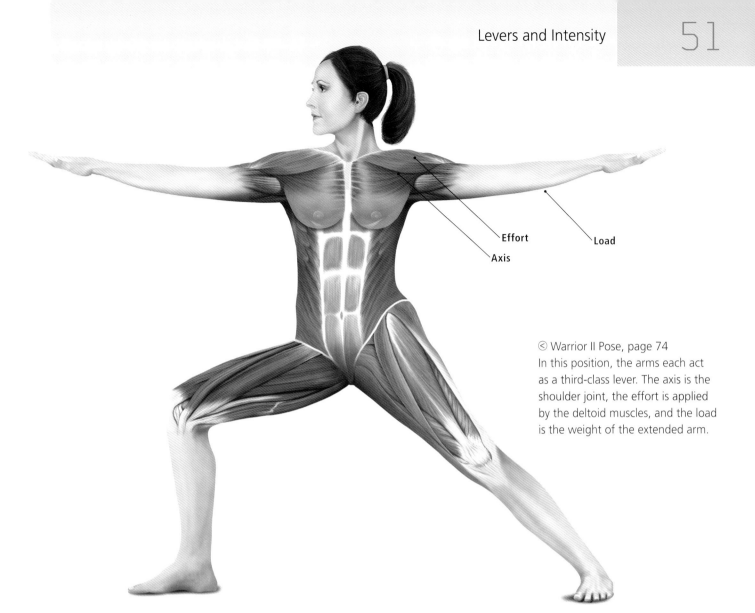

Effort

Load

Axis

⊘ Warrior II Pose, page 74
In this position, the arms each act
as a third-class lever. The axis is the
shoulder joint, the effort is applied
by the deltoid muscles, and the load
is the weight of the extended arm.

Second-class lever

In a second-class lever, the load is located between the
axis and the effort. A full push-up and the plank position
are examples of this. The ankles are the axis point, the
load is gravity, which is at its strongest at the center
of the body, and the effort is exerted predominantly
from the deltoids, the muscles of the shoulders.

Third-class lever

In a third-class lever, effort is applied between the load
and the axis. By extending the arms out to each side, as
in Warrior II Pose (page 74), the axis point is the shoulder
joint. Because we are not physically holding a weighted
object, the load is created by gravity and the weight
of the arm. The deltoids then exert the effort to keep
the arms raised.

Another example of this is Warrior III Pose (page 104).
The spine is in a forward flexion position and the axis point
is the sacroiliac joint at the bottom of the spine. Because
the arms are completely extended, the levers are long.
This means that the load (gravity) placed upon the body
is greater than if the hands were in front of the chest in
Prayer Position, for example. The muscles that support the
spine between the axis point (sacroiliac joint) and hands
then exert the effort—contract—to maintain the position
of the spine.

Modifications and Props

Yoga is a fundamentally accessible activity and can be practiced in a variety of settings and places, and it does not require much in the way of specialist equipment. However, there are a number of basic props you can use to help you get the most from yoga. These can also help to make some asanas more attainable for those with limited mobility. Throughout the book we have provided suggestions for possible modifications to the asanas, with or without props.

Yoga mat

A nonslip yoga mat is especially useful for standing poses where the feet are wide apart and there is a risk of slipping. They also act as padding for sitting and lying poses. Using a mat can also improve your sense of spatial awareness.

Yoga block

These are often used in sitting poses to elevate the hips and move the lower back into a neutral alignment. For example, when in a Seated Forward Bend (page 124), if there is tightness in the lower back or hamstrings, the pelvis sometimes tilts back. By placing a yoga block underneath the hips, the hips can tilt forward a little so the weight is directly on the seat bones, thereby straightening the spine.

Yoga brick

A yoga brick is often used to place the hand on if it does not reach the floor. In Revolved Triangle Pose (page 66), for example, the left hand (when turning to the right) needs to be in contact with either the floor or a yoga brick to maintain stability. A yoga brick can also be used in a more supportive manner, such as being placed under the sacrum in Shoulder Bridge Pose (page 168) to support the lower spine or under the top of the head when in a Wide-Leg Forward Bend (page 114) to support the neck.

Yoga strap

A yoga strap, depending on how it is used, can either assist in stretching muscles farther or can support the body. To stretch the muscles more deeply in a Seated Forward Bend (page 124), for example, a yoga strap can be placed around the balls of the feet, increasing the resistance and so encouraging the ankle joint to stretch more intensely. The hamstring and calf muscles also stretch more in this instance. Adversely, a yoga strap placed around the lower back, inner thighs, and ankles while in Cobbler's Pose (page 136), will let the legs and hips relax while still being supported by the yoga strap.

⊘ Seated Forward Bend, page 124
This position can be modified with the help of a yoga strap placed around the balls of the feet to create a more intense stretch.

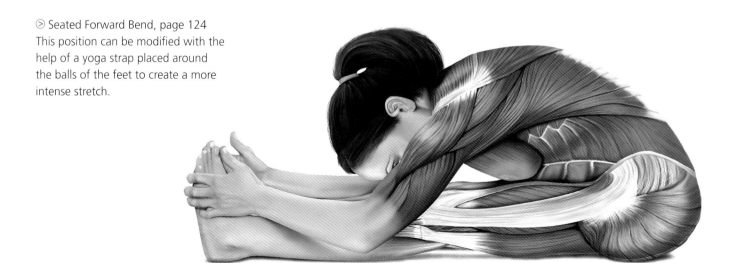

Blanket

A blanket can be used to provide padding for the body. For example, it can be placed underneath the hips in Boat Pose (page 128), or under the feet and ankles in Cobbler's Pose (page 136). It can also be used to cover the body in relaxation simply to provide warmth.

Wall

While not strictly a prop, a wall can be useful in learning poses that require a good deal of balance, such as Headstand Pose (page 180) or Half Moon Pose (page 100), because the wall can support the body and give the person a sense of correct alignment. Some wide-leg forward bends can also be practiced with the hands on a wall and the spine parallel to the floor instead of placing the hands to the ground.

Chair

Using a chair can be useful for those with limited mobility. For example, if moving to and from a sitting position on the ground is not possible, a spinal twist can be performed sitting on the chair with the feet on floor. The torso can then simply rotate to one side, with the left hand on the right knee and the right hand on the seat of the chair next to or behind the hips, before repeating on the other side.

ⓥ Yoga mats, bricks, and a yoga strap are shown below. Yoga bricks, often used to rest the hands on, are smaller than yoga blocks, which can be placed beneath the hips during sitting poses.

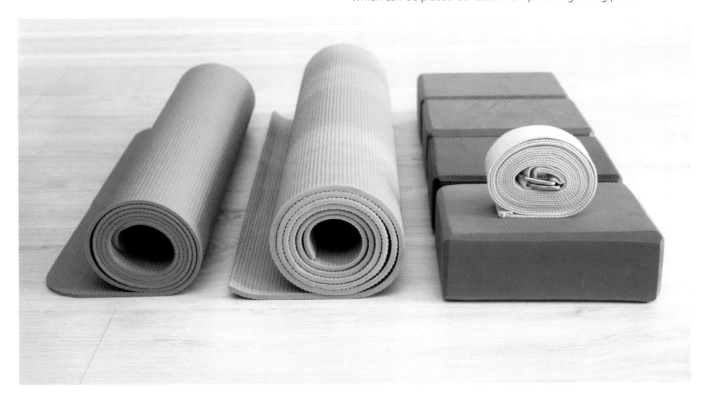

Starting Poses

There are four starting poses used throughout this book, and they are explained below. You will be referred back to one of these at the beginning of most asanas.

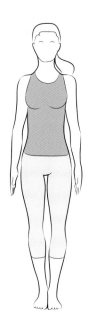

Mountain Pose
Tadasana

This is the foundation for all standing poses. Breathe steadily and stand upright with the arms by the sides and the feet together. Lift and spread the toes to help create a wide, solid base. Contract your thigh muscles so your kneecaps rise slightly, and draw the tailbone toward the floor to encourage neutral alignment of the pelvis and lumbar spine. Lift your sternum slightly, broadening the collarbone, and draw the shoulder blades downward. Elongate the neck so that the crown of the head rises toward the sky and the chin is parallel to the ground.

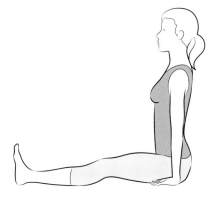

Staff Pose
Dandasana

Begin in a sitting position with the legs extended in front of the torso. The spine is perpendicular to the ground and the upper body is extending upward through the crown of the head. The palms of the hands are on the ground on each side of the body, in-line with the hips, with the shoulders rolling back and down. The legs are pressing together, and the toes are pointing upward with the feet in a neutral position. The abdominal muscles are contracting lightly to support the spine and the chin is level with the ground.

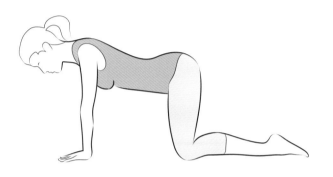

Box Pose

Begin on the hands and knees, with the thighs at righ angles to the back, and the arms perpendicular to the ground. Make sure the knees are set directly below the front of the hips and there is a space in between the knees. Align the shoulders directly over the elbows and wrists, and spread out the fingers and thumbs. Position the entire spine, including the neck, parallel to the ground. The eyes should be looking at the floor with the crown of the head pointing directly forward.

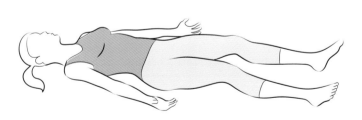

Corpse Pose
Savasana

This may look like a simple relaxing pose, done in between or after an asana, but it requires considerable concentration that develops through continued practice. It is practiced lying on the back with the legs straight and the feet hips' width apart. The feet should fall out gently to each side, with the arms resting alongside the body, slightly separated from the body, palms facing upward. Stretch through the body and draw the shoulder blades gently toward one another so the sternum lifts slightly. Start to breathe deeply, and slowly watch the breath. If this asana is being used for final relaxation, stay here for several minutes.

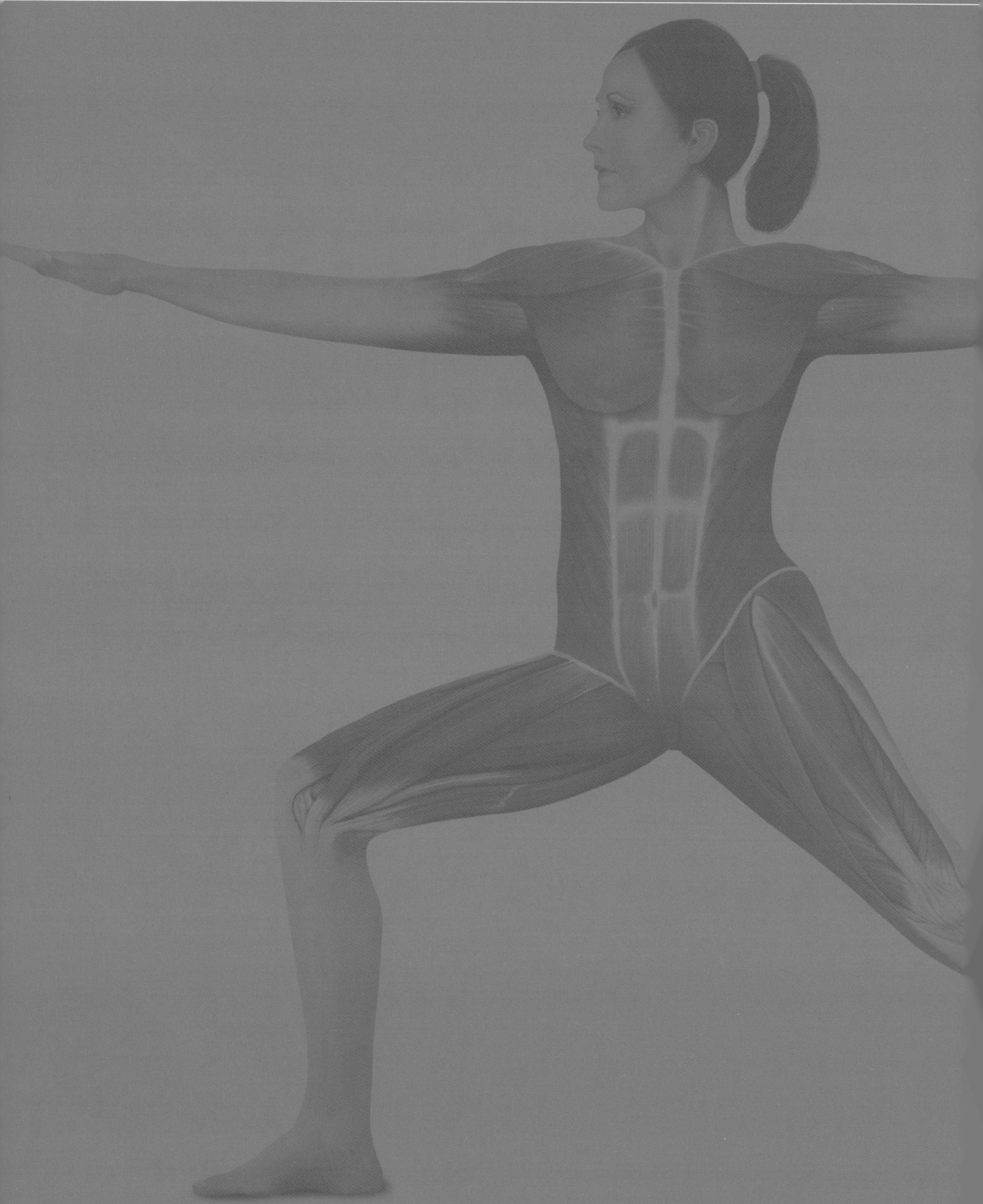

Standing Poses

Most yoga sequences involve standing poses, and these often make up a considerable part of a balanced hatha yoga practice. This is largely due to their effectiveness in warming up the muscles of the body and the ligaments and tendons of the joints, helping to prepare for asanas that stretch them more deeply while reducing the risk of injury. Longer term benefits include increased overall strength, flexibility, and stability, in particular, of the ankles, hips, and knees.

It is advisable that beginners in yoga focus mainly on standing yoga asanas to improve flexibility and posture of the spine to create a good physical foundation before the move on to the more challenging asanas.

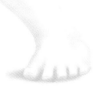

Chair Pose

Utkatasana

Chair Pose, also known as Fierce Pose, is a powerful asana that mimics sitting on a chair. It strengthens the whole body, in particular, the back, legs, and all the major joints of the body. To achieve this position, the hip flexors contract and shorten while the quadriceps lengthen, creating a slight forward tilt of the pelvis. The shoulder and upper back muscles work to raise the arms and draw the shoulder blades down. The larger muscle groups of the back then assist in maintaining the extension of the arms and the spine.

In this squatlike position, the shoulders, hips, knees, and ankles are all strengthened. For this reason, Chair Pose is useful to those who need to build up their strength before practicing stronger standing asanas, and it can be useful to practice when recovering from knee and ankle injuries, because it builds stability in these joints. In addition, because Chair Pose utilizes several muscles at the same time, the heart rate is increased, resulting in improved circulation and stamina.

Level

Beginner

Benefits

This asana strengthens all the major joints, including the shoulders, hips, knees, and ankles. It also improves stamina and muscle endurance.

Caution

People with lower back injuries or high blood pressure should exercise caution when attempting this pose.

Modifications and props

To lower the intensity of the pose, reduce the bend of the knees, and instead of extending the arms upward, place the hands in front of the chest in Prayer Position.

Position the feet hips' width apart if balance is an issue, but be careful to keep the knees in-line with the ankle joints.

Try to

Draw the pelvis downward as the knees bend, maintaining a neutral position through the lumbar spine and an even weight through the feet.

Press the legs together to create a sense of strength through the lower body.

Draw the shoulders down, away from the head, to create space across the shoulders.

Try not to

Do not round the spine in any way, including overarching through the lumbar spine. Instead, draw the coccyx down toward the ground.

If the spine moves into a concave position when the arms are raised, move the arms slightly wider than shoulders' width apart. This will help to make sure there is neutral alignment of the spine.

How to do it

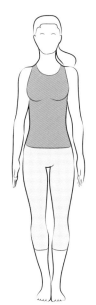

⊘ **Step 1**

Begin in Mountain Pose (page 54).

Step 2 ⊘

Press the feet and legs together and exhale while bending the knees so that the legs adopt a squat position. Spread the toes and make sure the heels remain on the ground, with the weight evenly distributed through the feet. The chin should be parallel to the ground and the arms by the sides.

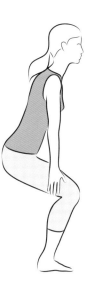

⊘ **Step 3**

On an inhale, sweep the arms upward so they are in-line with the ears and shoulders' width apart. The fingers and thumb of each hand should be closed together, not splayed. Now draw the shoulder blades down away from the head to create space across the top of the shoulders. Draw the coccyx downward to help elongate the lumbar spine region, and contract the lower abdominal muscles to assist in supporting the lower back. Lift the sternum and chin a little to create a sense of lift through the upper body, and breathe steadily.

Chair Pose

Utkatasana

In Chair Pose, there are many muscle groups working concentrically, eccentrically, and as fixators. The rectus femoris and the iliopsoas contract concentrically, helping to stabilize the pelvis. The erector spinae and quadratus lumborum lengthen eccentrically to allow for the flexion of the spine, before fixating it in extension. The knees are partly flexed, shortening the hamstrings. The deltoids fixate the arms overhead while the triceps maintain the extended position of the elbows. The dorsiflexion of the feet occurs when the tibialis anterior and gastrocnemius shorten concentrically and the soleus muscles contract eccentrically. The abdominal muscles, in particular, the rectus and transversus abdominis, act as stabilizers of the torso.

muscle activity

prime mover

1 Rectus femoris
2 Iliopsoas
3 Adductor longus
4 Pectoralis major and minor
5 Anterior deltoids
6 Lower trapezius
7 Erector spinae
8 Triceps
9 Latissimus dorsi

antagonist

10 Rhomboids
11 Quadratus lumborum
12 Rectus abdominis
13 Vastus lateralis
14 Vastus intermedius
15 Vastus medialis
16 Gluteus maximus

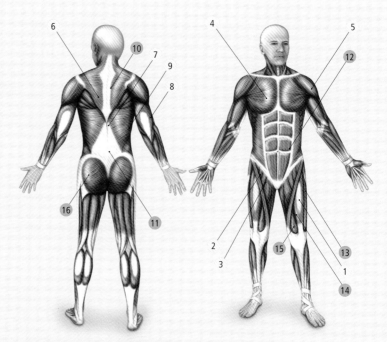

(7 beneath thoracolumbar fascia; 14 beneath rectus femoris)

spine

The pelvis is in an anterior tilt position, with the spine moving into extension at the final phase of the asana. The spine extends forward, moving in a sagittal plane from a medial lateral axis.

Anatomy of the pose

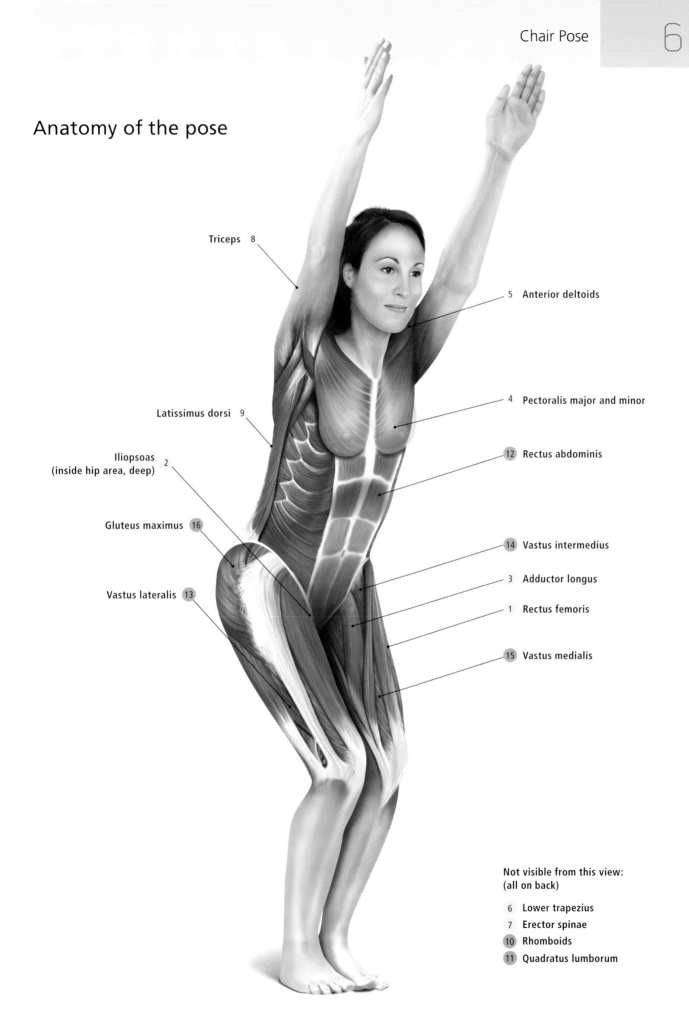

Triceps 8

5 Anterior deltoids

4 Pectoralis major and minor

Latissimus dorsi 9

12 Rectus abdominis

Iliopsoas
(inside hip area, deep) 2

Gluteus maximus 16

14 Vastus intermedius

3 Adductor longus

Vastus lateralis 13

1 Rectus femoris

15 Vastus medialis

Not visible from this view:
(all on back)

6 Lower trapezius

7 Erector spinae

10 Rhomboids

11 Quadratus lumborum

Triangle Pose

Trikonasana

Triangle Pose is a basic yoga posture that is commonly practiced in all styles of yoga. It stretches all the major joints, including the spine, shoulders, and hips. The spine will be in a deep side bend with the legs apart, so the body creates several triangles, the lines of which are strong and straight. This results in an intense stretch of several major muscles groups. The inner thigh of the front leg and outer thigh of the back leg are stretched, as are the hamstrings of both legs. The weight of the upper body is mainly over the front leg, so the back leg, foot, and lower back muscles have to work hard to maintain the body's balance. With the spine positioned in a deep side bend, the oblique abdominal muscles shorten on the right side of the torso and lengthen on the left side, increasing the overall strength of the core area. The arms are stretched away from the body and extended in opposite directions, with the right hand resting lightly on the ground behind the middle of the lower leg.

Level

Beginner

Benefits

This asana stretches and strengthens the legs; in particular, the muscles around the knees, ankles, hips, groin, and the hamstrings are all worked. It also opens the shoulders and chest.

Triangle Pose can help alleviate back pain by mobilizing the spine and stretching the surrounding muscles.

Caution

Due to the side bend of the lumbar spine, those with lower back injuries and/or conditions should practice this asana with caution.

Triangle Pose should be modified for those with neck injuries or groin strain.

Modifications and props

For back injuries, bend the right knee slightly and/or rest the left hand behind the lower back, so the back of the hand is against the back of the lumbar region.

For neck injuries, keep the chin in-line with the sternum (instead of looking upward).

⊘ Try to

Press firmly through both feet to work both legs equally.

Contract the abdominal muscles to support the lumbar spine, especially when moving in and out of the posture.

Move the left shoulder and hip back slightly, so the left shoulder stacks on top of right and the chest area feels open.

⊗ Try not to

Do not let the spine pass lower than parallel to the upper body, because this will mean length in the upper body will be lost. Instead, lengthen from the coccyx to the crown of the head.

Visualize a wall to the front and one behind. Stack the shoulders and hips so they do not touch the imaginary walls.

How to do it

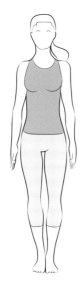

⊙ **Step 1**

Begin in Mountain Pose (page 54).

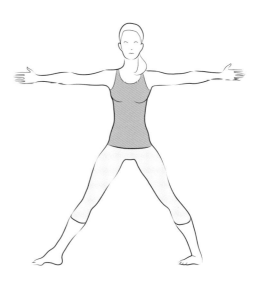

⊙ **Step 2**

Step the feet apart about 5 ft. (1.5 m) and extend the arms to each side so that they are parallel to the floor. Extend into the fingertips while drawing the shoulder down, and check that the feet are aligned under the wrists. Turn the left toes in forty-five degrees and the right foot out ninety degrees. The heels should be in-line with one another.

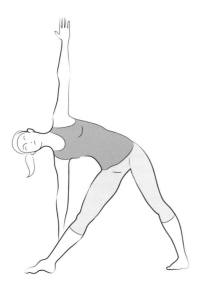

⊙ **Step 3**

Draw the spine upward and, with the arms still parallel to the floor, move the spine into a side bend, so that the mid- and upper torso are parallel to the ground. Be sure the arms are perpendicular to the ground, with the right hand resting lightly on the ground behind the middle of the tibia. Reach the left arm directly upward.

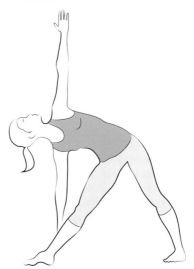

⊙ **Step 4**

Now move the left shoulder and hip back slightly and tuck the right hip under a little. This will create more of a stretch along the left side of the torso. Rotate the neck to rest the gaze toward the left hand.

Triangle Pose

Trikonasana

To allow for the deep sideways bend of the spine in Triangle Pose, the iliopsoas, gluteus minimus, piriformis, and quadratus femoris of the right leg have to externally rotate the femur to create the space in the right hip joint for the right ilium bone to laterally tilt. It is this action that lets the hamstrings lengthen, the gluteus maximus and hip flexors and quadriceps extend the legs, and the adductors and abductors lengthen. The lengthening through the right side is increased via an eccentric contraction of the gluteus medius and peroneus longus when the outer left foot presses firmly in to the ground. The obliques lengthen eccentrically on the left side while concentrically contracting on the right side, and the mid-deltoids abduct the arms away from the medial line, while the triceps extend the elbows. The scapulae are retracted toward the spine while the lower trapezius draws them away from the head. The sternocleidomastoid externally rotates the neck.

muscle activity

prime mover

1 External and internal obliques
2 Quadratus lumborum
3 Gluteus minimus
4 Piriformis
5 Quadratus femoris
6 Quadriceps
7 Triceps
8 Deltoids (midsection)
9 Sternocleidomastoid

antagonist

10 Rectus abdominis
11 Iliopsoas
12 Peroneus longus
13 Trapezius

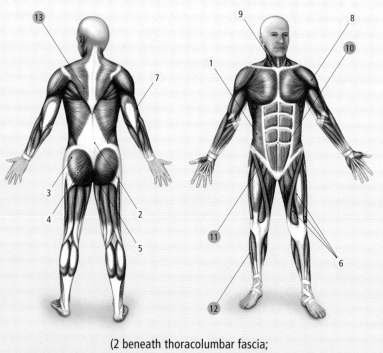

(2 beneath thoracolumbar fascia;
4 and 5 beneath gluteus maximus)

spine

The spine is in right lateral flexion, moving in a frontal plane from a sagittal axis. The pelvis is in a lateral tilt to the right.

Anatomy of the pose

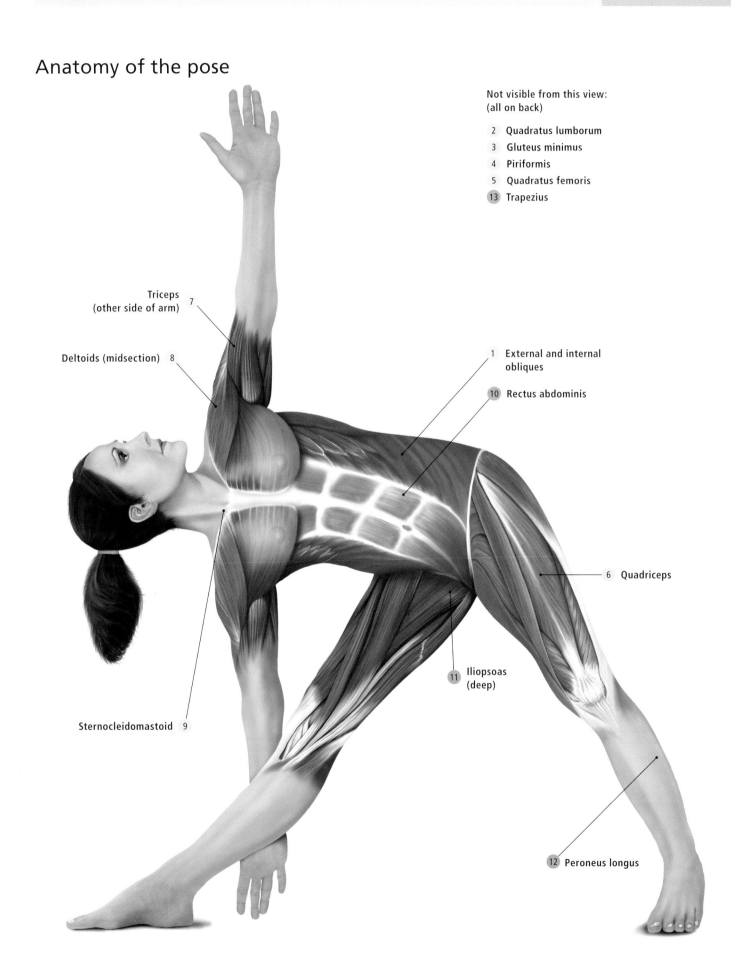

Not visible from this view:
(all on back)

2 Quadratus lumborum
3 Gluteus minimus
4 Piriformis
5 Quadratus femoris
13 Trapezius

Triceps
(other side of arm) 7

Deltoids (midsection) 8

1 External and internal
obliques

10 Rectus abdominis

6 Quadriceps

Iliopsoas
11 (deep)

Sternocleidomastoid 9

12 Peroneus longus

Revolved Triangle Pose

Parivrtta Trikonasana

This is a complex asana that improves flexibility and stability of all the major joints, in particular, the hips, and the ability of the torso muscles to rotate the spine. It is especially effective for improving posture, energy levels, and function of the internal organs, in particular, the digestive system. It is also effective in improving balance and awareness of space. The lower body will be required to act as a strong foundation; the quadriceps will be worked and the hamstrings stretched, so the spine can flex forward. The spine can then twist freely while the major muscle groups of the back, including the latissimus dorsi and the oblique abdominal muscle groups, stretch and provide stability simultaneously.

When the spine moves into Revolved Triangle Pose, it is in a rotated forward-bend position. While this is generally beneficial, the spine can become vulnerable to injury if the person pushes past their natural range of movement. Be careful to allow the muscles to stretch and release slowly.

Level

Intermediate

Benefits

This asana stretches and strengthens the hips, hamstrings, and calf muscles, and it opens the shoulders and chest to facilitate better breathing. Lower back pain is reduced and balance and stability of the entire body is improved.

Caution

People with lower back injuries and/or back conditions should practice this asana with caution. Revolved Triangle Pose should be modified for those with neck injuries, groin strain, or low blood pressure.

⊕ Modifications and props

If the hand does not comfortably reach the floor, place a yoga brick underneath it. This will help maintain even length through each side of the torso, helping to stretch the spine.

If the torso does not rotate completely to the right, keep the chin in-line with the sternum to avoid neck injury. Position the feet in a slightly diagonal stance if it is difficult to align the pelvis correctly.

⊘ Try to

Lower the spine, so it is parallel to the ground, and stretch all the way to the crown of the head. This will create space along the spine and enable better breathing.

Press the outer edge of the left foot down and contract the quadriceps muscles on both legs strongly to increase the sense of balance and stability in the lower body.

Rotate the upper body slowly, moving the right hip back a little at the same time, to create space in the hips.

⊗ Try not to

Avoid resting heavily on the left hand. The left hand should rest lightly on the ground, making sure the muscles around the waist support the lumbar region.

Try not to let the right shoulder drop forward; instead, draw the right shoulder back directly in-line with the left shoulder. This opens the chest and neck area.

How to do it

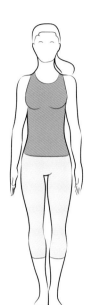

◁ Step 1

Begin in Mountain Pose (page 54).

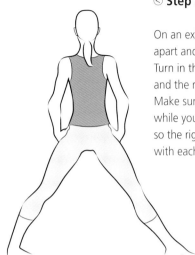

◁ Step 2

On an exhale, step the feet about 3 ft. (1 m) apart and place the hands on the hip bones. Turn in the left foot forty-five degrees to the right and the right foot ninety degrees to the right. Make sure the heels are aligned. Breathe steadily while you turn the torso and hips to the right, so the right and left front hip bones are in-line with each other.

◁ Step 3

Place the right hand to the lower back and extend the left arm directly upward. Press firmly into the feet and contract the thigh muscles. Inhale, extending the spine upward, then exhale while reaching the spine and left arm forward until they are parallel to the ground.

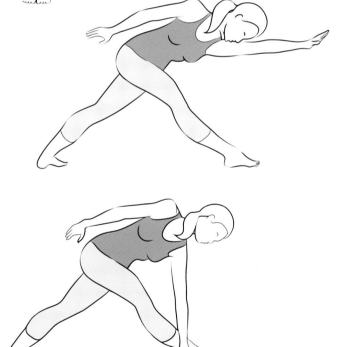

⌃ Step 4

Inhaling, reach the left hand to the floor to the outside of the right foot. Keep pressing firmly into the edge of the back foot. Now begin to exhale and rotate the torso from the navel, so that the right shoulder stacks on top of the left shoulder. The neck should be parallel to the ground.

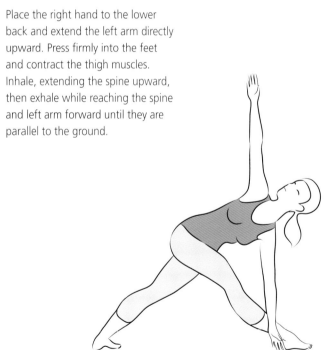

⌃ Step 5

Keep breathing deeply and move the right side of the hip bone back a little and extend the right arm upward, with the palm of the hand facing outward. The right and left arm should be in-line with one another. Keep the neck long and rest the gaze on the right hand.

Revolved Triangle Pose

Parivrtta Trikonasana

To allow for the initial forward flexion of the spine in Revolved Triangle Pose, the pelvis has to tilt forward. This is achieved by the hip flexors, which shorten concentrically with the iliopsoas stabilizing the pelvis. The hamstrings on the right and calf muscles (gastrocnemius and soleus) on the left lengthen eccentrically. The quadratus lumborum supports the lumbar region as it moves forward, and the spine rotates due to the activation of the internal and external oblique muscles. The back foot presses firmly into the ground as the peroneus longus lengthens, helping the right side of the pelvis to align with the left side of the pelvis, bringing it level to the ground. The deltoids work to abduct the arms, while the triceps extend the arms from the elbow. The lower trapezius muscles draw the scapulae down and away from the head, which lets the head turn more freely. The sternocleidomastoid externally rotates the neck.

muscle activity

prime mover

1 External and internal obliques
2 Sternocleidomastoid
3 Biceps femoris
4 Gluteus maximus and minimus
5 Triceps
6 Deltoids
7 Iliopsoas

antagonist

8 Adductors
9 Trapezius
10 Peroneus longus
11 Quadratus lumborum
12 Longissimus thoracis

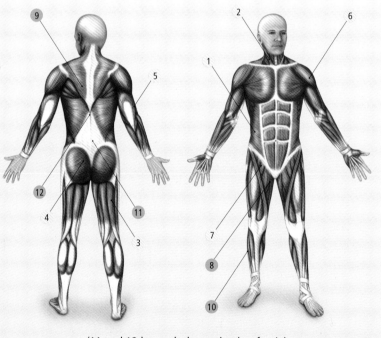

(11 and 12 beneath thoracolumbar fascia)

spine

The spine is in forward flexion and is rotated. It moves initially in a sagittal plane from a frontal axis, before rotating in a transverse plane. The pelvis is in an anterior tilt position.

Anatomy of the pose

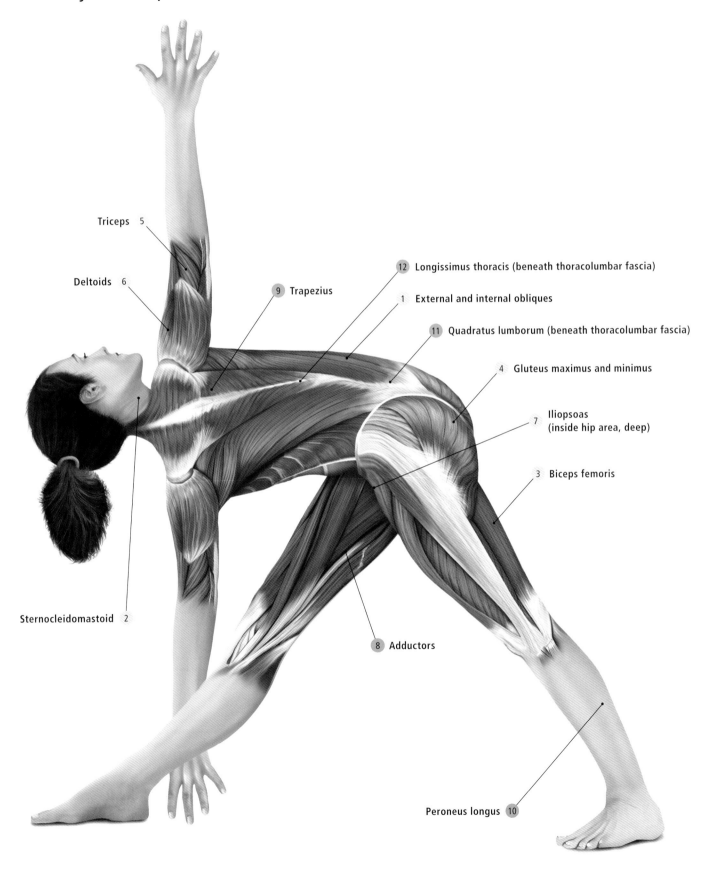

Triceps 5

Deltoids 6

9 Trapezius

12 Longissimus thoracis (beneath thoracolumbar fascia)

1 External and internal obliques

11 Quadratus lumborum (beneath thoracolumbar fascia)

4 Gluteus maximus and minimus

7 Iliopsoas (inside hip area, deep)

3 Biceps femoris

Sternocleidomastoid 2

8 Adductors

Peroneus longus 10

Warrior I Pose

Virabhadrasana I

Warrior I is an invigorating asana that is effective at increasing the range of movement of all the major joints. It encourages all the main muscle groups to work in synergy, which helps to open the hips and shoulders, strengthen the legs, arms, and back, and increase energy levels and mental focus.

The spine is in a slight backbending position, so it strengthens the extensors of the spine—mainly the erector spinae—and stretches the front of the upper body. The left leg is straight, so the hip flexors lengthen, while the right leg is bent and works powerfully with the quadriceps and adductors, which hold its position. This action of the legs helps to stretch and strengthen both sides of the hips and creates a strong foundation. The chest and front of the shoulders are open so the arms can reach directly upward. This creates a stretch and sense of lift through the entire upper body. Warrior I Pose can be practiced within Sun Salutation sequences or as part of a standing sequence.

Level

Intermediate

Benefits

Warrior I is an energizing asana that increases the heart rate and, thus, improves stamina. It stretches and strengthens the hip flexors, opens the chest and shoulders, and works the muscles of the back.

Caution

People with lower back injuries and/or back conditions should practice this asana with caution. Warrior 1 Pose should be modified for those with neck injuries, groin strain, or low blood pressure.

⊕ Modifications and props

If the hips are inflexible, move the right foot to the right by 2–4 in. (5–10 cm), to let the pelvis and lower back move more freely.

Separate the hands to shoulders' width apart if it is difficult to straighten the arms with the hands together.

For knee injuries, decrease the bend in the right leg; for neck injuries, look forward.

Try to

Press the edge of the left foot down firmly into the ground and align the right knee directly over the ankle; this will help prevent overstretching of the knee tendons.

Draw the scapulae downward to free up the neck.

Move the right front hip bone backward, and the left one forward.

Try not to

Never let the right knee move farther forward than directly over the ankle, and don't let the right thigh move inward, so the knee is no longer over the ankle.

Do not force the left front hip bone forward. The shoulders should not move upward. Do not overextend the lumbar spine.

How to do it

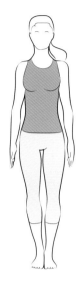

⊛ **Step 1**

Begin in Mountain Pose (page 54).

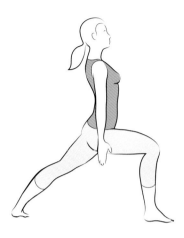

⊛ **Step 2**

On an inhale, take a big step backward, about 5 ft. (1.5 m), with the left foot. Turn the left foot out forty-five degrees, pressing the edge of the foot firmly into the ground. Exhale and bend the right knee to a right angle, so that the knee is aligned directly over the ankle. The ankles should be in-line with each other.

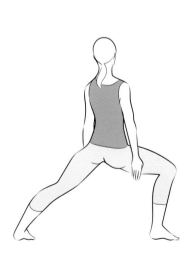

⊛ **Step 3**

Breathing steadily, press firmly into the feet and align the front of the rib cage and pelvis to face forward by moving the right hip back a little and the left hip gently forward. Extend the spine upward and gently contract the lower abdominal muscles to assist in supporting the lower back.

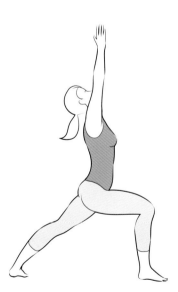

⊛ **Step 4**

Inhale and extend the arms directly upward, so they are in-line with the ears, and press the palms of the hands firmly together. Move the shoulders downward, away from the head. Lift the gaze up to the hands by moving the chin away from the chest, being careful not to overarch the lower back. Keep breathing steadily throughout.

Warrior I Pose

Virabhadrasana I

During Warrior I Pose, the right leg works powerfully, with the hip flexors and the hamstrings concentrically contracting. This moves the knee into a flexed position, with the quadriceps lengthening eccentrically and the adductors and gluteal muscles fixating the leg. The left leg is extended back due to a concentric contraction of the quadriceps and left gluteus maximus, while the sartorius and biceps femoris create an external rotation of the femur. The peroneus longus and soleus activate the edge of the left foot to supinate it slightly. This action helps to concentrically contract the quadriceps and stretch the front of the left hip.

The spine extends upward with the erector spinae shortening via a concentric contraction. The rectus abdominis and latissimus dorsi work to fixate this position. The deltoids initially extend the arms before fixating them in place, while the triceps extend the arms from the elbow. The trapezius draws the scapulae away from the head, allowing for the neck to extend more freely.

muscle activity

prime mover

1 Hamstrings
2 Quadriceps
3 Sartorius
4 Gluteus maximus and minimus
5 Trapezius
6 Erector spinae
7 Triceps
8 Deltoids
9 Hip adductors

antagonist

10 Iliopsoas
11 Latissimus dorsi
12 Rectus abdominis
13 Peroneus longus
14 Soleus

(6 beneath thoracolumbar fascia)

spine

The spine is in extension with slight external rotation of the left hip and left lumbar region. This asana moves in a sagittal plane with a slight movement in the transverse plane due to the external rotation of the left side. The spine moves from a frontal axis. The pelvis is in a slight anterior tilt.

Anatomy of the pose

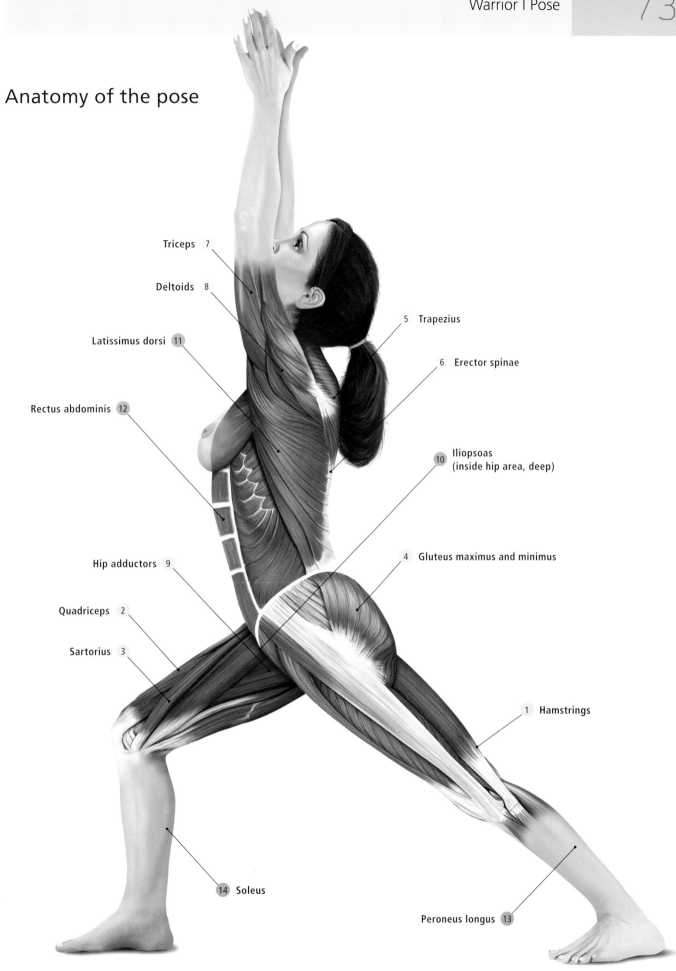

Triceps 7

Deltoids 8

5 Trapezius

Latissimus dorsi 11

6 Erector spinae

Rectus abdominis 12

Iliopsoas
10 (inside hip area, deep)

Hip adductors 9

4 Gluteus maximus and minimus

Quadriceps 2

Sartorius 3

1 Hamstrings

14 Soleus

Peroneus longus 13

Warrior II Pose

Virabhadrasana II

Warrior II is a standing asana that enhances posture, strength, stability, and concentration, and it can be an effective way to build a feeling of inner strength. It uses all the major muscle groups and opens the hips, chest, and shoulders while it strengthens the legs, arms, and back.

The right knee joint is bent, with the knee aligned over the ankle, and the left leg is straight; therefore, the quadriceps shorten on the left side and lengthen on the right side. This helps to open the front of the hips while the iliopsoas muscles help to stabilize the pelvis. The spine is extended upward and the chest area is broad and open. The arms are extended out strongly to each side, with the palms facing down, and the shoulder blades are drawing downward as the upper back muscles gently contract. The neck extensors help to turn the head so the gaze can rest to the right hand. With so many muscle groups working powerfully, the heart rate and circulation are increased, making this a particularly energizing asana.

Level

Beginner

Benefits

Warrior II Pose strengthens and stretches the legs, hips, and ankles and opens the chest area. It improves stamina by increasing the heart rate and circulation. The shoulders are also stretched and strengthened and mental focus is increased.

Caution

People with high blood pressure should be cautious with this asana.

Groin strain and knee and ankle injuries can also be exacerbated when the full asana is practiced; therefore, appropriate modifications should be used.

⊕ Modifications and props

For knee injuries, decrease the bend of the right knee; for lower back injuries, shorten the stance; and for sciatica, position the back foot at a ninety-degree angle.

For high blood pressure, position the hands in front of the chest in Prayer Position, so circulation is slowed.

⊘ Try to

Make sure the right knee is directly over the right ankle and the edge of the left foot is pressed down firmly, because this will help to stretch the left hip.

Elongate the spine to minimize pressure in the lower back, and keep the arms level, because this will help to strengthen the shoulders.

⊗ Try not to

Avoid stepping the feet too far apart, because this could overstretch the hips and affect balance. Conversely, if the stance is too short, the right knee can become overstretched, so do not let the right knee move past the ankle.

Do not let the shoulders move upward, because this will cause tension in the neck.

How to do it

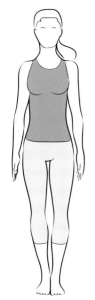

◁ Step 1

Begin in Mountain Pose (page 54).

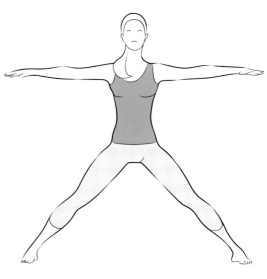

⌃ Step 2

On an exhale, move the feet about 5 ft. (1.5 m) apart; then, inhaling, extend the arms out to each side, so that they are parallel to the ground. Make sure that the heels are aligned with one another, and that the feet are aligned directly under the hands.

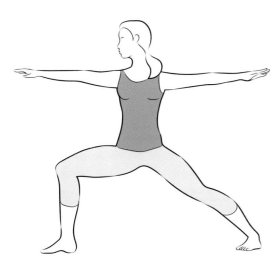

◁ Step 3

Turn the right foot out ninety degrees and the left foot in forty-five degrees, and align the right heel with the arch of the left foot. Then, exhale while bending the right knee, moving the leg into a right-angle position. Make sure the right knee is aligned directly over the right ankle. The left leg should remain straight and the thigh firm. Breathing evenly, press the outer left foot firmly into the floor and draw the coccyx downward to lengthen the lower back. The shoulder blades should draw downward and the arms should be strong. Rest the gaze toward the right hand, with the chin level to the floor.

Warrior II Pose

Virabhadrasana II

During Warrior II, the spine is in extension, initiated by the erector spinae, with the latissimus dorsi and rectus abdominis working as fixators. The arms are abducted away from the medial line of the body and are parallel to the floor with the hands in pronation. While the triceps contact concentrically to extend the arms from the elbows, it is the deltoids that hold the arms in place. The hamstrings of the right leg are shortening concentrically, creating flexion at the knee joint, and the quadriceps lengthen to let this movement occur. Conversely, the left leg is completely extended with the gluteal muscles and quadriceps activated concentrically and the hip flexors lengthened eccentrically. The sartorius and biceps femoris of the left leg are the hip flexors that externally rotate the thigh and hip to create a stretch across the front of the pelvis and in the adductors. It is the peroneus longus that lengthens as the outer left foot presses firmly in to the ground. The scapulae are retracted toward the spine while the trapezius draws them away from the head. The sternocleidomastoid rotates the head and neck.

muscle activity

prime mover

1 Hamstrings
2 Quadriceps
3 Adductors
4 Gluteus maximus and medius
5 Sartorius
6 Erector spinae
7 Triceps
8 Deltoids
9 Trapezius

antagonist

10 Latissimus dorsi
11 Rectus abdominis
12 Iliopsoas
13 Peroneus longus

(6 beneath thoracolumbar fascia)

spine

The spine is in extension, moving in a frontal plane from a sagittal axis.
The pelvis is in a neutral position.

Anatomy of the pose

Not visible from this view:

4 Gluteus maximus and medius (rear of leg)
6 Erector spinae (on back)
7 Triceps (rear of arm)
9 Trapezius (on back)
10 Latissimus dorsi (on back)

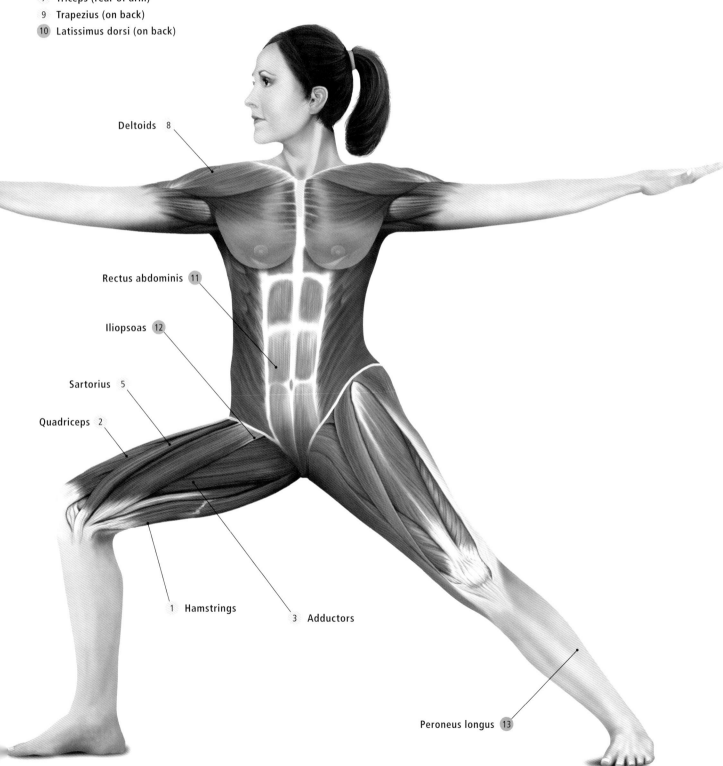

Deltoids 8

Rectus abdominis 11

Iliopsoas 12

Sartorius 5

Quadriceps 2

1 Hamstrings

3 Adductors

Peroneus longus 13

Extended Side-Angle Pose

Utthita Parsvakonasana

Extended Side-Angle Pose is a strong asana that works all the major muscle groups and requires considerable flexibility of the major joints, in particular, the hips and shoulders. For this reason, it is considered a "master posture."

With the left leg completely extended and the right knee flexed to a right angle, the legs create a strong foundation. The core muscles of the upper body work to hold the body in place. By reaching the left arm over to create a straight line, the entire left side of the body is stretched, increasing the flexibility of the rib cage. The flexibility of the lower back and hips can be increased by moving the outer left hip back a little. This creates a deeper stretch on the left side of the body; however, it can sometimes be too intense for beginners and should, therefore, be practiced with caution.

Level

Intermediate

Benefits

This asana strengthens and stretches the legs, hips, shoulders, and ankles.

It increases stamina by elevating the heart rate and improves respiration by stretching the lungs. Increasing the flexibility of the connective tissue of the rib cage allows for greater expansion and deeper breathing.

Caution

People with high blood pressure should be cautious with this asana.

Groin strain and knee and ankle injuries can also be exacerbated when the full asana is practiced; therefore, appropriate modifications should be used.

⊕ Modifications and props

For knee injuries, decrease the bend of the right knee. For lower back injuries and high blood pressure, shorten the stance and place the right forearm on the right thigh. For sciatica, position the back foot at a ninety-degree angle.

⊘ Try to

Make sure the right knee is directly over the right ankle and the edge of the left foot is pressed down firmly, because this will help to stretch the left hip.

Elongate the spine to minimize pressure in the lower back, and keep the arms level, because this will help to strengthen the shoulders.

⊗ Try not to

Try not to rest on the right hand or forearm.

How to do it

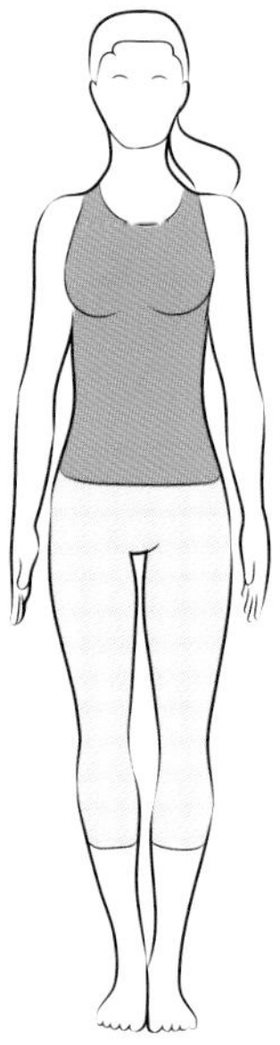

◎ **Step 1**

Begin in Mountain Pose (page 54).

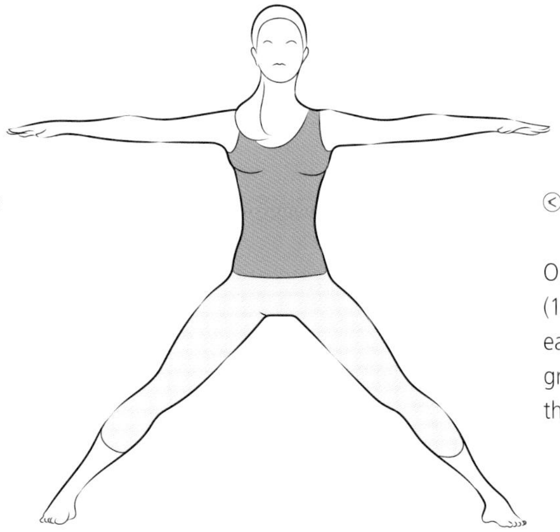

◎ **Step 2**

On an exhale, move the feet about 5 ft. (1.5 m) apart. Next, extend the arms out to each side, so that they are parallel to the ground. Make sure that the heels align and the feet are aligned directly under the hands.

Step 3 ⊗

Inhale while turning the right foot out ninety degrees and the left foot in forty-five degrees, and align the right heel with the arch of the left foot. Exhale and bend the right knee, moving the leg into a right-angle position. Make sure that the right knee is directly over the right ankle.

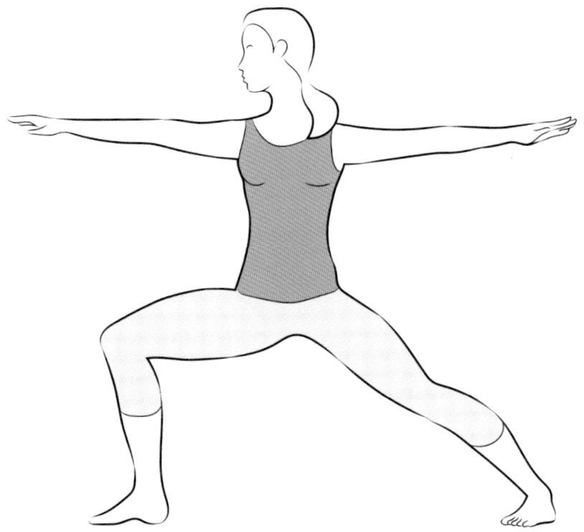

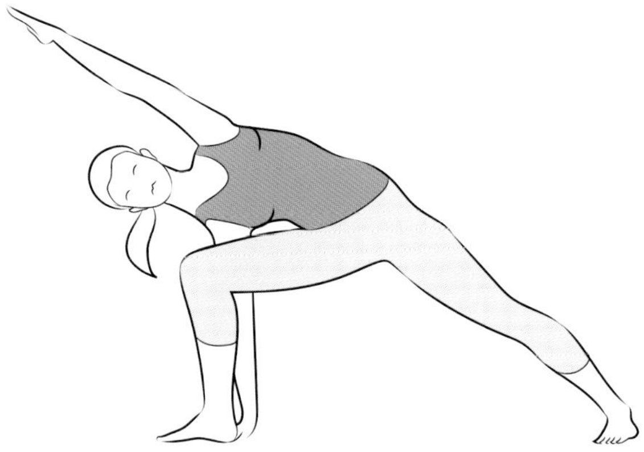

⌃ **Step 4**

Extend the torso to the right, placing the right hand on the ground behind the right leg. Inhale and extend the left arm up to align with the left ear, creating a long straight line from the edge of the left foot to the left fingertips. The palm of the left hand should be facing the ground.

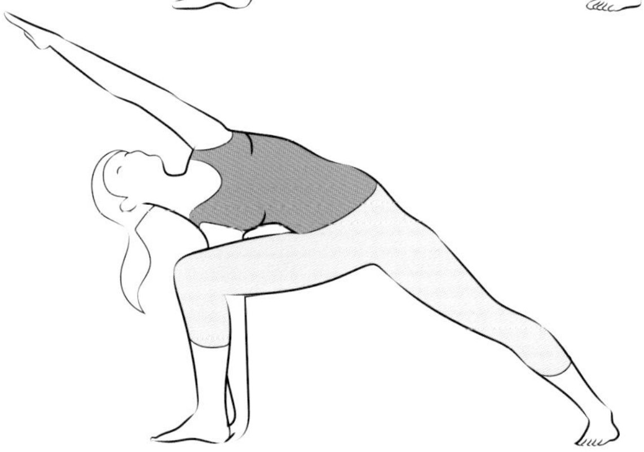

⌃ **Step 5**

Move the left hip back slightly as the right hip moves forward, increasing the stretch in the hips. Maintain the strength through the legs and abdominal muscles, so that the right arm does not have to support the posture. Bring the gaze to the left hand and breathe steadily.

Extended Side-Angle Pose

Utthita Parsvakonasana

To allow for the deep flexion of the right knee in Extended Side-Angle Pose, the hamstrings shorten and the quadriceps lengthen, while the adductors assist to hold the leg in position. The left leg is completely extended and the concentric contraction of the quadriceps is maximized by the peroneus longus lengthening and assisting to press the edge of the left foot in to the ground. The hip flexors, sartorius, and biceps femoris then externally rotate the left leg and hip slightly, helping to open the entire left side of the body. The hamstrings of the left leg now lengthen eccentrically.

The spine is in deep lateral flexion to the right, achieved by the obliques and quadratus lumborum on the right side of the body, as they contract concentrically. The latissimus dorsi and rectus abdominis then fixate the upper body in place. The arms are abducted away from the medial line by the deltoids, with the left arm extended over the head via a concentric contraction of the serratus anterior. The pectorals lengthen eccentrically. The scapulae are retracted toward the spine while the trapezius draws them away from the head. The sternocleidomastoid rotates the neck.

muscle activity

prime mover

1 Hamstrings
2 Quadriceps
3 Gluteus maximus and medius
4 Quadratus lumborum
5 Sartorius
6 Triceps
7 External and Internal obliques
8 Serratus anterior

antagonist

9   Latissimus dorsi
10 Rectus abdominis
11 Iliopsoas
12 Peroneus longus
13 Trapezius
14 Deltoids
15 Adductors

(4 beneath thoracolumbar fascia)

spine

The spine is in right lateral flexion, moving in a frontal plane from a sagittal axis.
The pelvis is in a lateral tilt to the right.

Anatomy of the pose

Not visible from this view:

3 Gluteus maximus and medius (rear of leg)
4 Quadratus lumborum (on back)
9 Latissimus dorsi (on back)
13 Trapezius (upper back)

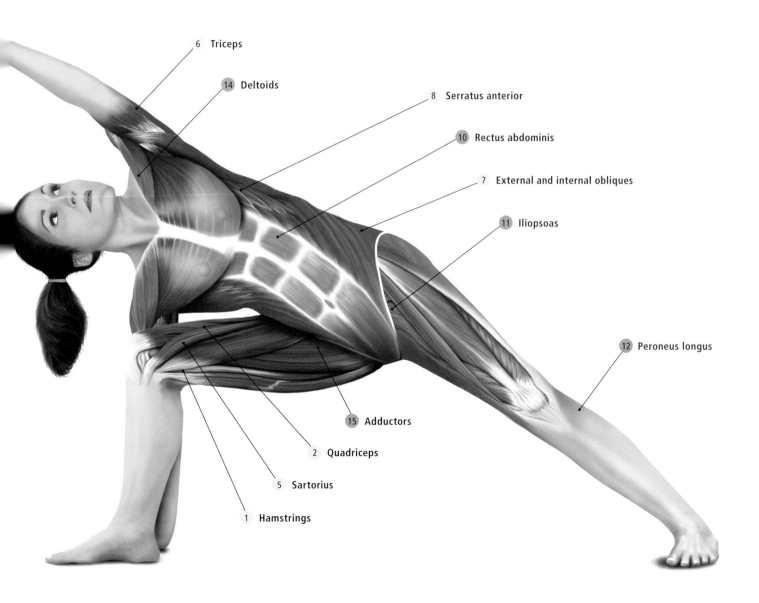

6 Triceps

14 Deltoids

8 Serratus anterior

10 Rectus abdominis

7 External and internal obliques

11 Iliopsoas

12 Peroneus longus

15 Adductors

2 Quadriceps

5 Sartorius

1 Hamstrings

Revolved Side-Angle Pose

Parivrtta Parsvakonasana

Revolved Side-Angle Pose is an asana that requires a great level of flexibility and strength. It is extremely effective in increasing the mobility of all the major joints and the entire spine, and it increases flexibility of the thoracic region in particular. The legs are worked hard and the front of the hips are stretched deeply, allowing for the pelvis to move into the correct alignment. The left leg is completely extended and the right knee is flexed to a right angle, creating a strong foundation for the upper body. The core muscles work powerfully to rotate the upper body, and as a result of this rotation the internal organs, including the digestive system, are stimulated, creating a detoxifying effect.

The flexibility of the spine and hips can be increased with a small external rotation of the right shoulder. This creates a deeper stretch on the right side of the body. However, this can be too intense for people with injuries and should be practiced with caution.

Level

Advanced

Benefits

This asana stretches the entire body and strengthens the legs, shoulders, and ankles. The hips, in particular, are stretched, while the heart rate is increased, improving respiration.

The rotation of the spine also momentarily compresses some of the internal organs, which stimulates digestion.

Caution

People with injuries to the vertebral disks should not practice this asana.

Those with other lower back issues or knee injuries should modify this asana.

⊕ Modifications and props

To modify this asana, place a brick under the left hand and place the right hand on the lower back; this will decrease the range of motion.

To decrease the rotation of the spine, place the left arm on the inside of the right leg.

⊘ Try to

Make sure the right arm is parallel to the ground and try to create as much length through the spine as possible before rotating the upper body.

Rest the left hand lightly on the ground and maintain strength through the legs and abdominal muscles.

Create a long straight line from the edge of the left foot to the right fingertips.

⊗ Try not to

Avoid resting heavily on the left hand, because this will build pressure in the wrist.

Avoid lifting the edge of the back foot from the floor and resting the upper body on the right thigh.

Do not strain the neck to look at the right hand. Instead, if uncomfortable, keep the chin in-line with the sternum.

How to do it

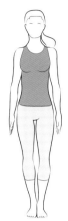

⊙ Step 1

Begin in Mountain Pose (page 54).
(Steps 1–3 viewed from front)

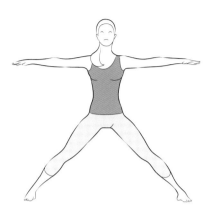

⊼ Step 2

Step the feet about 5 ft. (1.5 m) apart; then, on the next inhale, reach the arms out to each side, so that they are parallel to the floor.

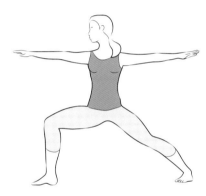

⊼ Step 3

Turn the right foot out forty-five degrees and the left foot in ninety degrees. Exhaling, bend the right leg to a right angle, aligning the knee over the ankle.

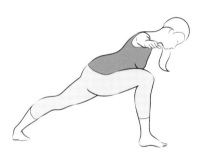

⊼ Step 4

(Steps 4–6 viewed from side)
Rotate the upper body to the right and extend the spine over the right thigh at the same time. Keep pressing the left foot firmly down onto the ground and sink the right hip back as the left hip moves forward a little. The arms should still reach out to each side.

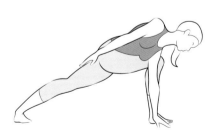

⊼ Step 5

Place the right hand on the lower back and, on an exhale, rotate the upper body deeply to the right, placing the left arm to the outside of the right leg, in-line with the lower leg and ankle. Once the left hand is on the ground, pause and inhale, and then, while exhaling, rotate farther, so that the right shoulder now aligns over the left shoulder.

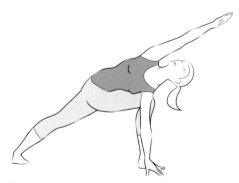

⊼ Step 6

Breathing steadily, extend the right arm upward, before exhaling as it extends over the head, so that it is in-line with the right ear. Really stretch from the edge of the left foot all the way to the fingertips on the right hand to get a deep stretch in the right side of the rib cage. Rest the gaze toward the right hand.

Revolved Side-Angle Pose

Parivrtta Parsvakonasana

In Revolved Side-Angle Pose, the left knee is flexed, with the hamstrings and hip flexors shortening concentrically and the quadriceps lengthening eccentrically. These actions are reversed on the right leg, with the hamstrings lengthening eccentrically and quadriceps shortening, leading to full extension of the knee. The adductors work to stabilize both legs, while the iliopsoas supports the pelvis. There is also an inward rotation of the right leg as the upper body rotates to the left. The entire spine, but particularly the thoracic spine, deeply rotates due to a strong concentric contraction of the latissimus dorsi and internal and external obliques. To support this position, the quadratus lumborum supports the lumbar region while the rectus abdominis assists to fixate the upper body. The triceps extend the arms from the elbows while the deltoids and serratus anterior work to extend the left arm over the head. The trapezius retracts the scapulae and the sternocleidomastoid externally rotates the neck.

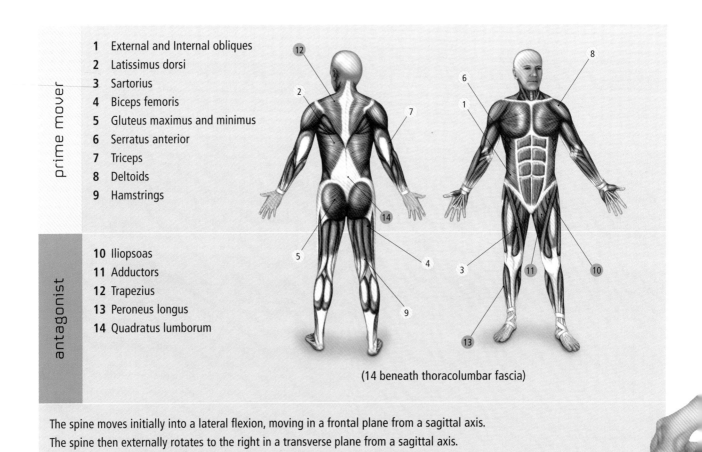

prime mover

1   External and Internal obliques
2   Latissimus dorsi
3   Sartorius
4   Biceps femoris
5   Gluteus maximus and minimus
6   Serratus anterior
7   Triceps
8   Deltoids
9   Hamstrings

antagonist

10 Iliopsoas
11 Adductors
12 Trapezius
13 Peroneus longus
14 Quadratus lumborum

(14 beneath thoracolumbar fascia)

The spine moves initially into a lateral flexion, moving in a frontal plane from a sagittal axis.
The spine then externally rotates to the right in a transverse plane from a sagittal axis.
The pelvis is in an anterior tilt.

Anatomy of the pose

Not visible from this view:

2 Latissimus dorsi (on back)

11 Adductors (inner thigh)

12 Trapezius (upper back)

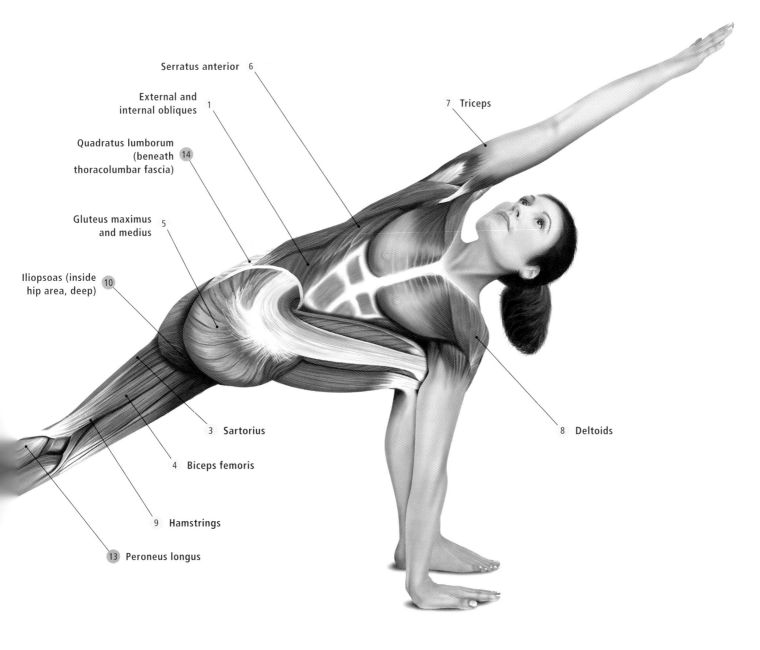

Serratus anterior 6

External and
internal obliques 1

Quadratus lumborum
(beneath 14
thoracolumbar fascia)

Gluteus maximus
and medius 5

Iliopsoas (inside
hip area, deep) 10

7 Triceps

8 Deltoids

3 Sartorius

4 Biceps femoris

9 Hamstrings

13 Peroneus longus

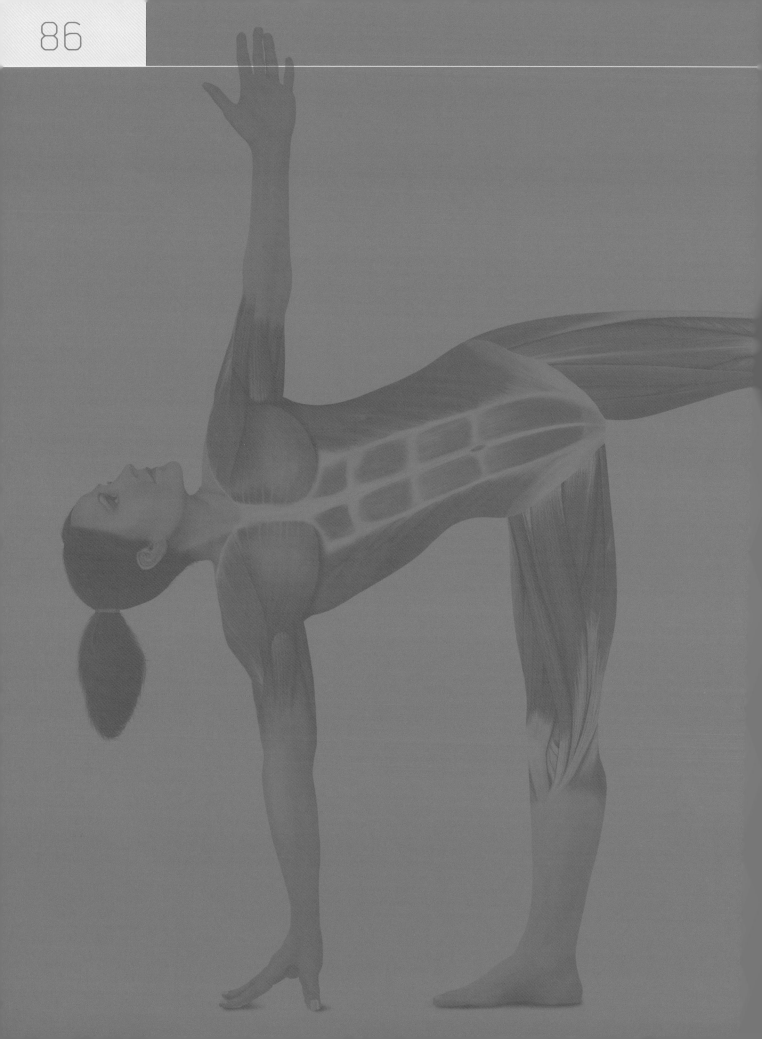

Standing Balancing Poses

These asanas are often practiced once the body is warm. They greatly improve the strength of the knees and ankles. This is largely due to the small stabilizing muscles and connective tissues in and around the joints becoming active in stabilizing the knee and ankle, so the participant does not lose their balance. Furthermore, all asanas that involve an element of balance will greatly improve mental focus and clarity, because concentration is required to practice these asanas effectively.

Tree Pose

Vrksasana

Tree Pose is a balancing asana that greatly improves the strength, flexibility, and stability of all the major joints. The left leg is straight, with the knee joint completely extended, and the quadriceps work hard to hold the leg in place. The adductors and gluteal muscles also assist with this action. The hip flexors lift the right thigh toward the upper body and move it outward from the hip joint, so the right foot can rest on the left inner thigh. The hip flexors contract to help support the pelvis and lumbar region during these actions. The spine is elongated and, because there is no movement forward, backward, or to either side in this asana, it is in a neutral position. The arms reach overhead with the hands pressed firmly together, giving a sense of lift and lightness, and the sacral region is drawn downward to counteract possible overextension of the lumbar region when the arms are extended. Maintaining this stance helps to slow down erratic or fast-pace breathing, lowers the heart rate, and calms the nervous system. It creates a sense of stillness in mind and body.

Level

Beginner

Benefits

Tree Pose improves postural awareness and alignment.

It encourages the person to focus on their breathing, which, in turn, improves mental focus and rejuvenates the mind and body.

Caution

For those with high blood pressure or ankle or knee injuries, proceed with caution and modify the asana. People with sciatica should also proceed with caution.

⊕ Modifications and props

For high blood pressure, place the hands in Prayer Position in front of the chest.

For ankle or knee injuries, place the raised foot on the inside of the ankle of the opposite leg, with the toes touching the floor, to provide more support.

For those who struggle to balance, practice Tree Pose with a wall for support.

Try to

Be sure both legs feel strong and keep the hips level with one another, so each side of the lower back are working equally. Keep the chin level to the floor and the shoulders drawing downward.

Feel a sense of lightness through the body by reaching upward and elongating the spine.

Make sure the right foot is placed on the left inner thigh; avoid placing the foot on the inside of the knee joint.

⊗ Try not to

Try not to lift the shoulders toward the head when the arms are raised. If the shoulders are lifting, separate the hands instead and move the shoulder blades down.

Try not to bend the left knee and instead focus on straightening the knee and contracting the quadriceps.

Anatomy of the pose

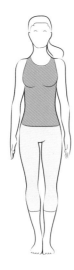

⌃ Step 1

Begin in Mountain Pose (page 54).

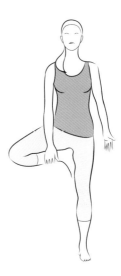

⌃ Step 2

Transfer the weight to the left foot and contract the muscles of the left thigh. Now, press down into the left foot, exhale, and place the right foot on the inside of the left inner thigh, placing the right hand around the right ankle to move the foot into position. The right knee should be bent and pointing out to the side and the hips level with one another. Press the right foot firmly into the left inner thigh and relax the toes.

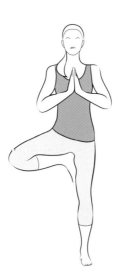

⌃ Step 3

Inhale while lifting the hands to chest height, pressing them together in Prayer Position. The elbows should be pointing down toward the ground and the shoulders should be relaxed. Pause and breathe.

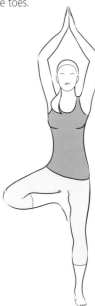

⌃ Step 4

Inhale again while extending the arms upward, until the hands are directly over the head, still in Prayer Position. The elbows should be slightly bent and the shoulders drawn downward. Straighten the spine upward, relax the face, and look forward with the chin level to the floor.

Tree Pose

Vrksasana

Throughout Tree Pose, the spine is in a neutral position and is supported by the major muscles surrounding the thoracic and lumbar region. These include the erector spinae and abdominal muscles, which are contracted isometrically. The arms are extended overhead when the deltoids contract concentrically. The triceps also work concentrically while the biceps femoris lengthen eccentrically to extend the arms from the elbows, and the trapezius muscles retract the scapulae away from the head. The quadriceps of the left leg are contracting concentrically to completely extend the knee, while the stabilizers around the knees and ankle work hard to fixate these joints in place. The gluteal and abductors also work powerfully to stabilize the leg. The right femur is externally rotated from the hip joint when the gluteus minimus and hip flexors, sartorius, and biceps femoris shorten concentrically and the hamstrings shorten to flex the right knee. The iliopsoas shortens concentrically on the right side and fixates on the left side.

muscle activity

prime mover

1 Iliopsoas
2 Quadriceps
3 Sartorius
4 Biceps femoris
5 Gluteus minimus
6 Deltoids
7 Triceps

antagonist

8 Gluteus maximus
9 Trapezius
10 Serratus anterior

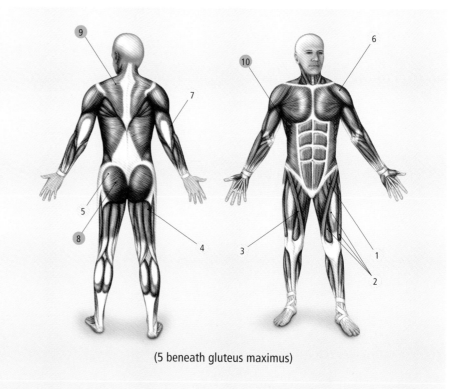

(5 beneath gluteus maximus)

spine

The spine is in a neutral position. The pelvis is also in a neutral position.
Therefore no movement occurs in a plane or around an axis.

Anatomy of the pose

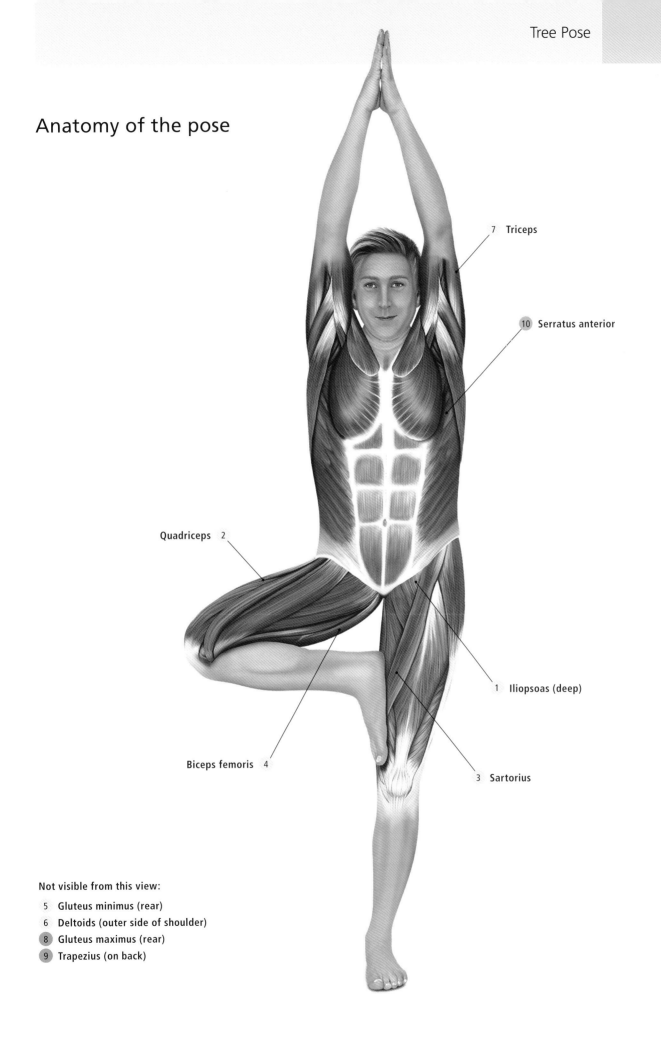

7 Triceps

10 Serratus anterior

Quadriceps 2

1 Iliopsoas (deep)

Biceps femoris 4

3 Sartorius

Not visible from this view:

5 Gluteus minimus (rear)

6 Deltoids (outer side of shoulder)

8 Gluteus maximus (rear)

9 Trapezius (on back)

Eagle Pose
Garudasana

Eagle Pose is an invigorating asana that improves balance and coordination. It stretches the upper back and shoulders and strengthens all the major joints of the body. Due to the balancing elements of this asana, the knees and ankles are greatly strengthened, because they work hard to stabilize themselves. The hips, knees, and elbows are all flexed, causing a momentary restriction of the blood flow through the joints, which then results in improved circulation when the pose is released.

When the hands move away from the face and the shoulder blades move away from one another, the upper back muscles are stretched. The extensors of the spine contract, so the upper body remains upright. The legs are pressed together, strengthening the adductors and quadriceps and stretching the outer thigh. This, in turn, helps to maintain good alignment of the kneecap, which benefits the knee joint. Eagle Pose also stretches the gluteal muscles, which helps ease lower back pain, and it stretches the muscles that surround the sciatic nerve, helping to ease some cases of sciatica.

Level

Beginner

Benefits

This pose strengthens the ankles, knees, and hips, and stretches the shoulders. It improves core stability and can ease pain in the lower back.

Caution

Those with knee, ankle, and shoulder injuries should practice with caution.

People with low blood pressure should practice this asana gently and be careful not to overexert themselves.

⊕ Modifications and props

For knee and/or ankle injuries, place a yoga brick under the toes of the right foot or place the toes on the floor to offer support to the injured joint.

If the shoulders are stiff or injured, place the right arm under the left and rest the backs of the hands together, instead of the palms.

Try to

Draw the shoulders downward and align the hands and wrists directly over the elbows.

Move the knees to the center line of the body, so they are aligned over the ankles, and press the legs together to improve stability.

Try not to

Try not to tighten the shoulders by letting the scapulae lift.

Do not lean forward; instead, extend the spine upward.

Do not force the right foot behind the left calf muscle, because this may injure the knee; rest the foot gently on the left lower leg instead.

How to do it

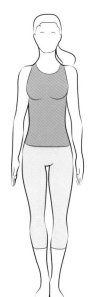

⊚ Step 1

Begin in Mountain Pose (page 54).

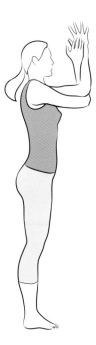

Step 2 ⊚

Inhale and stretch the arms straight out in front of the body, so they are parallel to the ground. While exhaling, sweep the right arm underneath the left arm, bending the elbows at the same time. Now inhale and press the palms of the hands together. The fingers and thumbs should be pointing upward and the forearms should be perpendicular to the floor.

Step 3 ⊚

Exhaling, move into a squat position by pressing the legs and feet together and bending the knees, keeping the heels firmly on the ground and extending the spine upward. The thighs should be pressing together and the pelvis tilting forward slightly. Draw the abdominal muscles in toward the spine.

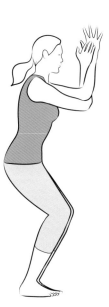

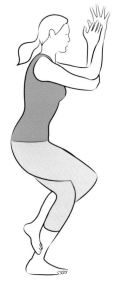

⊚ Step 4

Keeping the left leg bent, inhale while lifting the right leg up and over the left leg, placing the right thigh on top of the left thigh. Tuck the right foot behind the left lower leg so the right toes are pointing downward. The crown of the head should be drawn upward, extending the spine. The gaze should be directly forward and the chin level to the floor. Breathe steadily.

Eagle Pose

Garudasana

In Eagle Pose, the hamstrings are concentrically contracted and the quadriceps lengthened eccentrically, causing flexion at the knee. The iliopsoas, sartorius, and biceps femoris all shorten, causing flexion at the hips. This, in turn, moves the spine into forward flexion before the erector spinae shortens concentrically, creating a slight extension in the lumbar spine. The right ankle joint is plantar flexed, while the left ankle is dorsiflexed and the adductors work hard to press the thighs together. This results in the femurs both rotating internally. The gluteal muscles work to stabilize the hips, and the abdominal muscles—mainly the rectus abdominis—assist to fixate the upper body in place. The pectorals and anterior deltoids draw the arms toward one another, while the trapezius and rhomboids draw the scapulae downward, creating a stretch across the upper back and neck.

muscle activity

prime mover

1 Gastrocnemius
2 Sartorius
3 Biceps femoris
4 Iliopsoas
5 Deltoids
6 Erector spinae
7 Adductors
8 Pectoralis major and minor

antagonist

9 Soleus
10 Gluteus maximus and medius
11 Trapezius
12 Quadriceps

(6 beneath thoracolumbar fascia)

spine

The spine is in extension, moving in a sagittal plane from a frontal axis.
The pelvis is in an anterior tilt.

Anatomy of the pose

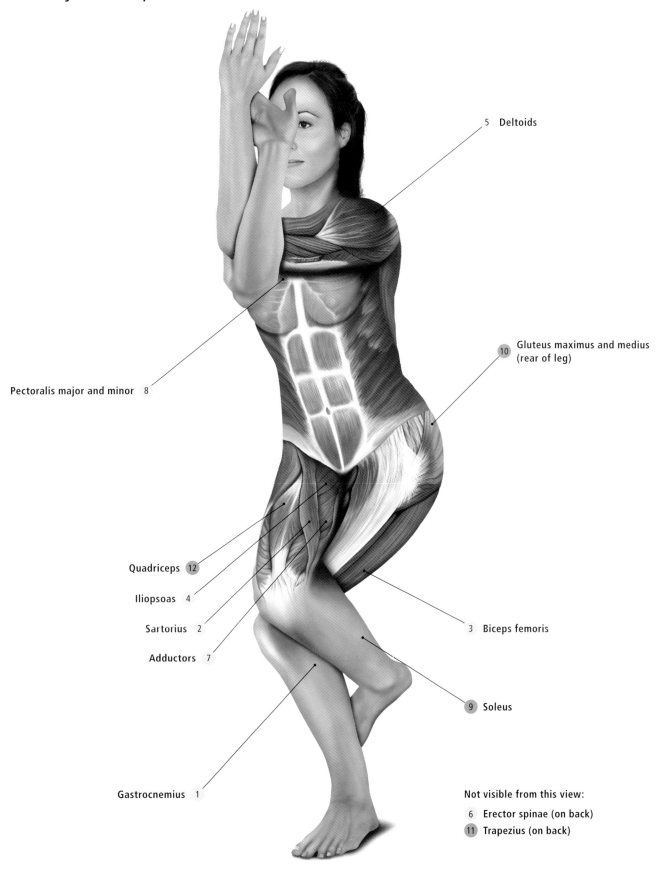

5 Deltoids

10 Gluteus maximus and medius (rear of leg)

Pectoralis major and minor 8

Quadriceps 12

Iliopsoas 4

Sartorius 2

Adductors 7

3 Biceps femoris

9 Soleus

Gastrocnemius 1

Not visible from this view:

6 Erector spinae (on back)

11 Trapezius (on back)

Dancer's Pose

Natarajasana

Dancer's Pose is an energizing asana that requires complete mental focus. It is a strong balancing asana that uses every muscle group in the body, and it is considered a backbending asana due to the deep extension of the spine. Overall benefits of Dancer's Pose include increased circulation and improved respiratory function, meaning general stamina is, in turn, greatly improved.

The standing leg stays completely straight and supports the body's weight, while the other leg kicks back, with the knee flexed. This kicking action makes sure that the pelvis tilts forward, and the upper body also moves forward, with the spine moving into a backbending position. For this action to occur, the right shoulder and right hip have to rotate outward, creating a deep stretch in these joints. The ankle and knee of the left leg work hard to stabilize the body, improving their strength and stability. As a result of all the major muscle groups working in synergy in this way, core stability is also greatly improved.

Level

Intermediate

Benefits

Dancer's Pose improves stamina. It stretches and strengthens all the major joints, particularly the hips and shoulders, and greatly improves mental focus.

Flexibility of the spine and core stability is also greatly improved.

Caution

This asana is intensive and so should be modified for those with high or low blood pressure.

For people with lower back injuries, there should be minimal rotation in the pelvis to avoid excessive pressure on the spinal disks.

⊕ Modifications and props

For blood pressure or lower back issues, modify Dancer's Pose by focusing more on elongating the spine and reaching the left arm upward instead of extending the spine and left arm forward.

If it is difficult to bend the knee, place a yoga strap around the ankle and hold the strap with the right hand.

⊘ Try to

Elongate the spine, creating a sense of space in the upper body.

Keep the standing leg completely straight to protect the knee joint and improve balance.

Let the right arm relax as the right leg kicks back, because this will help the shoulder joint to stretch.

⊗ Try not to

Try not to lower the left arm past parallel; instead, keep it on the same level as the eyeline and reach forward strongly.

Avoid rotating the right hip too powerfully, because this may compress the lower back. Instead, let the right hip move toward the ground a little.

How to do it

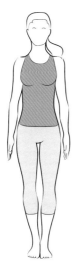

⌃ Step 1

Begin in Mountain Pose (page 54).

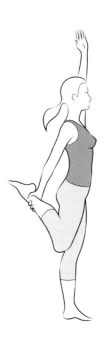

⌃ Step 2

Rotate the right arm until the inner elbow and palm of the hand are facing outward. Now transfer the weight to the left leg and bend the right knee, lifting the right foot toward the right gluteal muscle. Place the right hand firmly around the inside of the right ankle. Inhale and extend the left arm directly upward at the same time, so the left upper arm is in-line with the left ear.

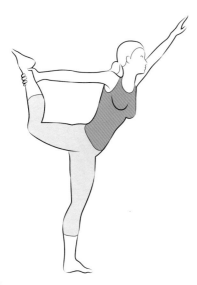

⌃ Step 3

Press down into the left foot and keep the left leg completely straight by strongly contracting the thigh muscles. Exhale while kicking the right foot back and upward so the upper body tilts forward and the left arm reaches forward, too. Breathe evenly as the spine extends forward. There should be a sense of lifting and length through the upper body.

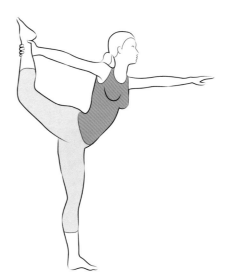

⌃ Step 4

Exhaling, kick the right foot backward more powerfully, so that the extension of the spine is increased. The right leg should now kick upward with the right hip and shoulder turning out to the right. The left arm should reach forward with the hand in-line with the gaze, which is directly forward. The chin should be level to the ground.

Dancer's Pose

Natarajasana

There are several muscle groups working differently during Dancer's Pose. The hamstrings of the right leg shorten to create the flexion at the knee, while the quadriceps and hip flexors lengthen eccentrically. The posterior deltoid and rotator cuff of the right shoulder externally rotate the right arm. The triceps work concentrically to extend both arms, with the deltoid of the left shoulder contracting isometrically to hold the arm in place and the pectoral muscles working concentrically to assist. The left leg is completely extended, with the quadriceps contracting concentrically and the hamstrings working to fixate this action. The pelvis is rotated anteriorly and the spine is extended in a backbending position, with the erector spinae shortening concentrically. The latissimus dorsi and rectus abdominis help to fixate the position of the spine.

muscle activity

prime mover

1. Quadriceps
2. Hamstrings
3. Erector spinae
4. Deltoids
5. Gluteus minimus and maximus

antagonist

6. Rectus abdominis
7. Pectoralis major and minor
8. Latissimus dorsi

(3 beneath thoracolumbar fascia)

spine

The spine is in extension, moving in a sagittal plane from a frontal axis.
The pelvis is in an anterior tilt position.

Anatomy of the pose

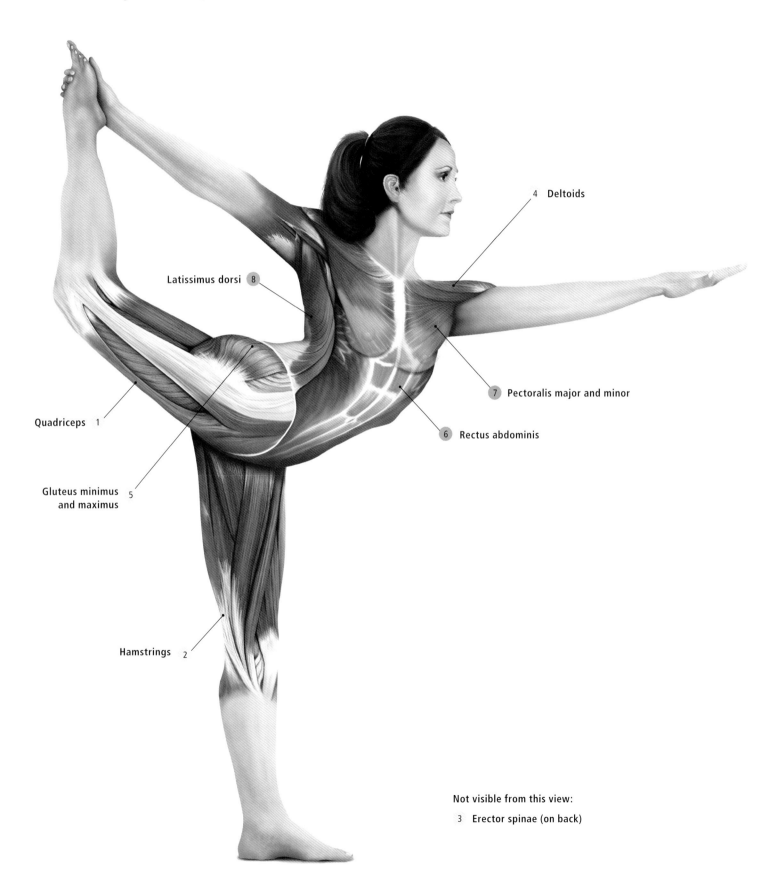

4   Deltoids

Latissimus dorsi   8

7   Pectoralis major and minor

Quadriceps   1

6   Rectus abdominis

Gluteus minimus
and maximus   5

Hamstrings   2

Not visible from this view:

3   Erector spinae (on back)

Half Moon Pose
Ardha Chandrasana

Half Moon Pose is a balancing asana that is especially effective in increasing the strength and stability of all the joints, in particular, the knees and ankles. Moving into this asana, the spine bends to the right side and the right knee is bent, allowing for the right hand to reach the floor just in front of the right foot. As the left foot lifts from the ground, both knees straighten and the legs work hard. All four corners of the standing foot are rooted to the ground, while the raised foot is in a neutral position. The spine elongates to create equal length on each side of the torso, and the abdominal muscles work powerfully to support the spine. The arms reach away from the body to create a long line from one hand to the other, stretching the chest and shoulders. The front of the hips and groin also stretch due to the outward rotation of the left hip. This rotating action should not be forced, however, because it can put unnecessary stress across the lower back joints.

Level

Intermediate

Benefits

This pose stretches and strengthens the hips while strengthening the ankle and knee joints. The shoulders and chest are stretched and core stability is greatly improved.

Because this asana requires good balance, concentration is also improved.

Caution

People with blood pressure issues or lower back injuries, especially spinal disk injuries, should modify this asana.

⊕ Modifications and props

If the right leg cannot be straightened when the right hand is on the ground, place a yoga brick under the right hand.

If the spine requires additional support, position the back of the body against a wall.

For neck injuries, keep the gaze directed toward the right hand.

For blood pressure issues, keep the left hand on the left hip.

Try to

Contract the leg muscles powerfully to help extend the knee joints.

Externally rotate the left side of the body back a little, so the joints are stacked in one line, creating space in the hips and shoulders.

Reach the arms and legs away from the center of the body to create space in the joints.

Try not to

Do not let the left leg drop lower than parallel to the floor; instead, create a long straight line from the left heel to the crown of the head.

Try not to drop the left shoulder and left hip forward and aim to open these joints by drawing the left side of the body backward.

How to do it

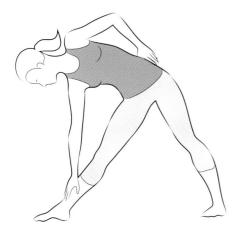

◁ Step 1

Begin in triangle pose to the right side. Now place the left hand on the left hip and the right hand on the right lower leg. The left shoulder and left hip are externally rotating and the crown of the head and neck are lengthening away from the body.

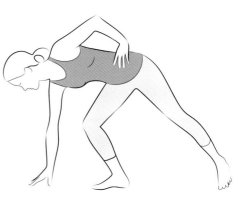

Step 2 ▷

Maintain steady breathing while transferring the body's weight onto the right leg and bending the right knee. Shorten the stance by moving the left foot in a little toward the right. Reach the right hand to the ground just to the side of the foot, in front of the toes. The right hand is now directly under the right shoulder and the body's weight is mainly on the right leg. The left leg is straight, with the foot hovering just above the ground.

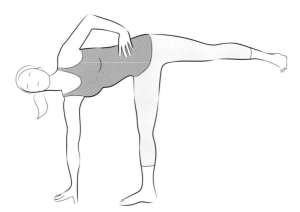

⋀ Step 3

Now straighten the right leg while inhaling and simultaneously raising the left leg parallel to the ground. Extend through to the left heel to straighten the left knee, pointing the toes forward. Contract the thigh muscles firmly and straighten the knees completely.

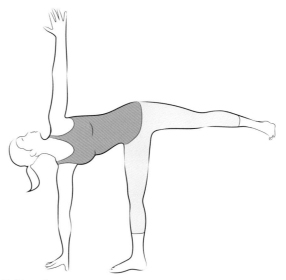

⋀ Step 4

Exhaling, rotate the left hip and left shoulder back slightly to increase the stretch through the left side of the body before extending the left arm directly upward. The arms should now create one long line. Keep the neck straight and move the gaze to the left hand.

Half Moon Pose

Ardha Chandrasana

Although the spine is laterally flexed to the right in Half Moon Pose, equal length through each side of the torso is required. This initially requires the oblique muscles on the right to contract concentrically as the spine moves into a side bend. The abdominal muscles, including the rectus abdominis, then work as fixators when the spine begins to elongate. The left oblique muscles contract to externally rotate the left hip and shoulders, moving them into a neutral position, while the quadratus lumborum supports the lumbar spine area. The quadriceps work concentrically to extend the knee joints, and the hamstrings lengthen eccentrically to allow for this movement. The gluteus maximus helps to extend the hips and the gluteus minimus helps to stabilize the pelvis while the abductor muscles move the right leg away from the medial line of the body. The standing leg is externally rotated by the quadratus femoris and sartorius hip flexor. The arms are initially externally rotated before being abducted away from the body by the deltoids. The triceps contract concentrically to extend the arms from the elbow joint. The left side of the sternocleidomastoid shortens concentrically to bring the gaze to the left hand.

muscle activity

prime mover

1 Sternocleidomastoid
2 Quadriceps
3 Gluteus maximus and medius
4 Internal and external obliques
5 Deltoids
6 Quadratus femoris

antagonist

7 Hamstrings
8 Quadratus lumborum
9 Sartorius

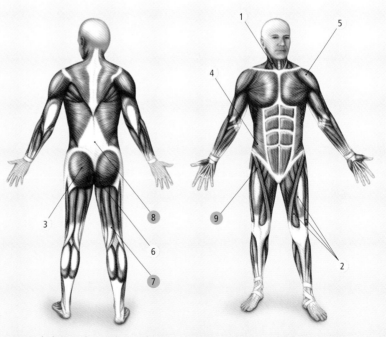

(6 beneath quadratus femoris; 8 beneath thoracolumbar fascia)

spine

The spine is in right lateral flexion, moving in a frontal plane from a sagittal axis.
The pelvis is in a lateral tilt to the right.

Anatomy of the pose

Not visible from this view:

3 Gluteus maximus and medius (rear of leg)
6 Quadratus femoris (beneath gluteus maximus)
8 Quadratus lumborum (on back)

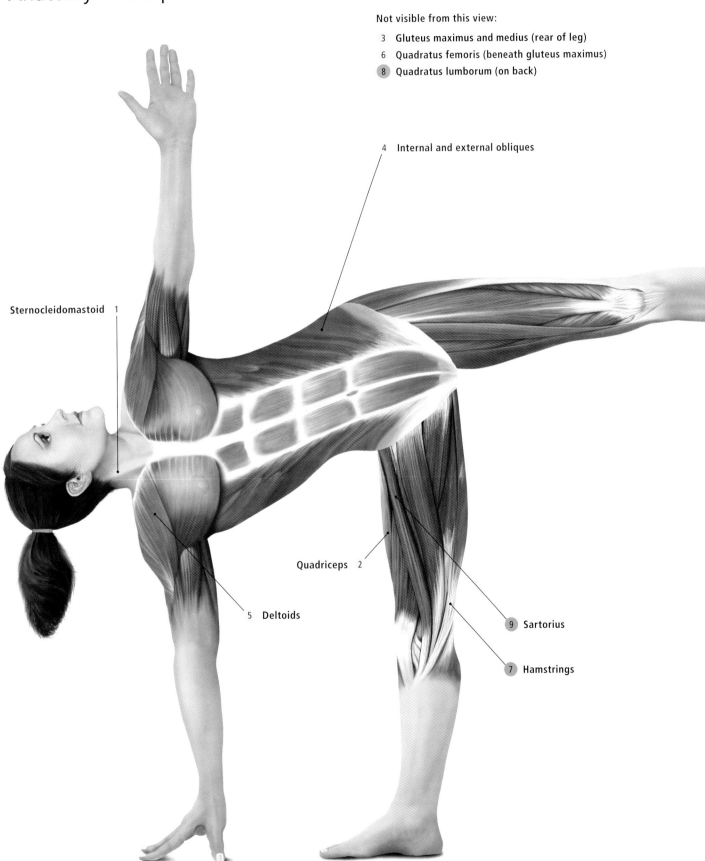

4 Internal and external obliques

Sternocleidomastoid 1

Quadriceps 2

5 Deltoids

9 Sartorius

7 Hamstrings

Warrior III Pose

Virabhadrasana III

Warrior III is considered one of the more challenging balancing poses. Due to the extension of the arms and legs, it requires strength from all the major muscles groups and is, therefore, particularly effective at building muscle endurance and aerobic stamina.

Initially, the arms are extended overhead from Mountain Pose, and the spine elongates to create space through the upper body. This action stretches the spine and helps to open the shoulder joints. The thigh muscles, mainly the quadriceps, contract powerfully, which helps to extend the knees, while the gluteal muscles extend the hips. This creates a long line from the feet to the hands and stretches all the joints, energizing the entire body. When the right leg steps forward, the spine is lowered parallel to the ground, so the muscles supporting the spine and shoulders have to contract powerfully to maintain the position. The quadriceps and hamstrings work even more powerfully, while the stabilizers of the ankle joints and the abdominal muscles work to maintain the person's balance.

Level

Intermediate

Benefits

This asana strengthens the entire body. It stretches the shoulders and gives the person a sense of length through the body.

Because of the intensity of this asana, aerobic and muscle endurance are greatly improved.

Caution

Because the arms and legs are completely extended, this asana works the lower back intensely and increases the heart rate. This asana should, therefore, be modified for those with lower back injuries or high or low blood pressure.

⊕ Modifications and props

For lower back injuries or blood pressure issues, postion the arms by the side of the body or place the hands in Prayer Position in front of the sternum.

The alignment of the body can also be modified by moving the spine and raised leg to a diagonal line instead of the lower body being parallel to the ground. This will minimize pressure on the lower back.

⊘ Try to

When reaching the arms overhead, try to lengthen and straighten the entire body.

Maintain the straight line through the body and contract the abdominal muscles to support the lumbar region.

The pelvis should be level to the ground when moving into the final position.

⊗ Try not to

Try not to lift the shoulders upward; focus on moving the shoulder blades down, away from the ears.

Avoid rotating the pelvis; instead, focus on maintaining a neutral alignment of the hips.

Avoid rounding the spine; instead, keep a straight line through the body, keeping the arms in-line with the ears.

How to do it

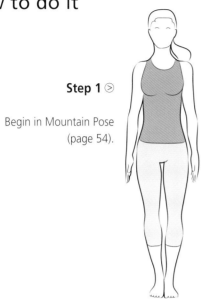

Step 1 ⊘

Begin in Mountain Pose (page 54).

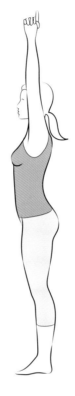

⊘ **Step 2**

Reach the arms out to each side and then extend them up overhead. Interlace the fingers firmly and extend the index fingers, pressing the heels of the hands together firmly. Move the shoulders down, away from the ears. Now press the legs firmly together and elongate the entire body, stretching the back muscles and shoulders. Draw the lower front rib cage in and draw the coccyx down toward the ground.

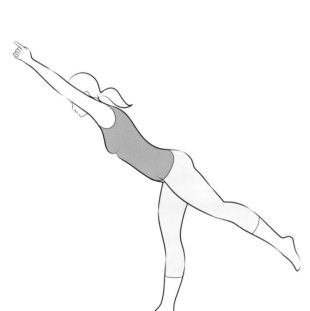

⊘ **Step 3**

Step the right leg forward about 2 ft. (60 cm) and transfer the body's weight to the right leg. Then, keeping the left leg straight, lift the left foot from the ground and extend the left leg backward as the spine and arms extend forward. The left leg, spine, and the arms now create a long diagonal line.

Step 4 ⊘

Keep the knees straight and contract the thigh and gluteal muscles strongly. Extend into the left heel and point the toes downward while keeping the hips parallel to the ground. The spine and arms should be reaching forward with the crown of the head pointing forward, creating a long straight line from the left heel to the fingertips. Lower the gaze to the ground without dropping the head down.

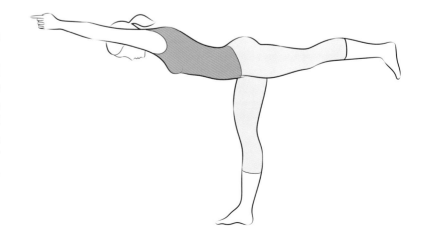

Warrior III Pose

Virabhadrasana III

In Warrior III, the deltoids extend the arms overhead. The arms are internally rotated by the teres major and pectoral muscles and held in place by the serratus anterior. The triceps contract concentrically to extend the elbow joints. The scapulae are initially rotated before the trapezius muscles move the scapulae down and away from the head. The spine is extended and supported by the erector spinae, quadratus lumborum, and latissimus dorsi. The rectus abdominis isometrically contracts to fixate the spine. The right hip is flexed due to a concentric shortening of the hip flexors, while the left hip joint is extended by the gluteus maximus and the knees are extended by quadriceps. Both of these muscle groups are in a concentric contraction. The tibialis anterior muscles shorten and the soleus and gastrocnemius muscles lengthen to create a dorsiflexion at the ankles.

muscle activity

prime mover

1 Erector spinae
2 Quadriceps
3 Gluteus maximus
4 Tibialis anterior
5 Trapezius
6 Triceps
7 Deltoids
8 Teres major

antagonist

9 Latissimus dorsi
10 Rectus abdominis
11 Quadratus lumborum
12 Serratus anterior

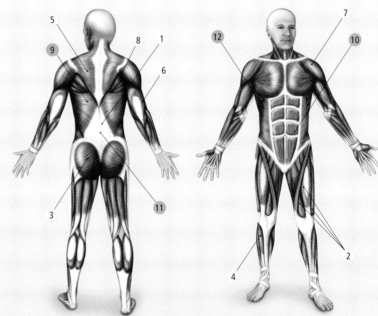

(1 and 11 beneath thoracolumbar fascia)

spine

The spine is extended in a sagittal plane from a frontal axis.
The pelvis is in an anterior tilt position.

Anatomy of the pose

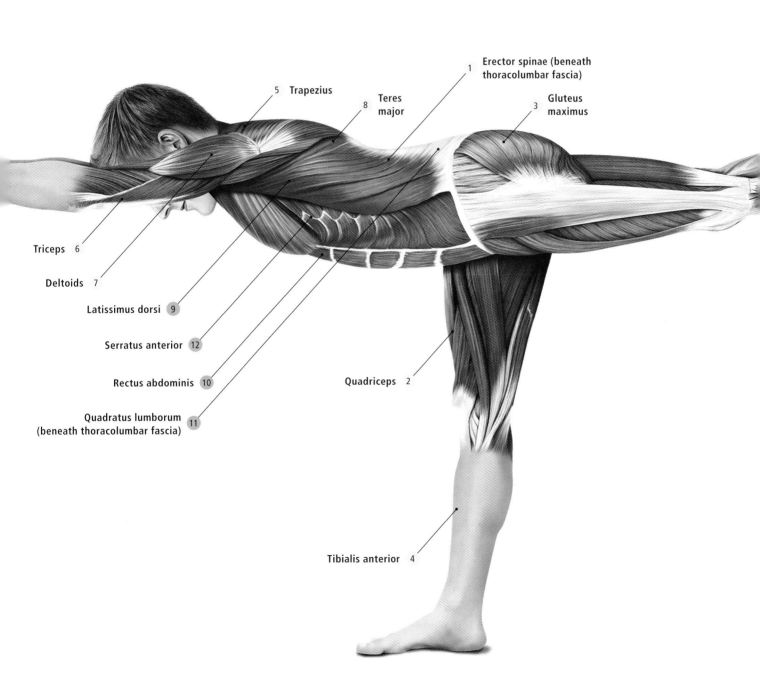

Erector spinae (beneath thoracolumbar fascia) 1

5 Trapezius

Teres major 8

Gluteus maximus 3

Triceps 6

Deltoids 7

Latissimus dorsi 9

Serratus anterior 12

Rectus abdominis 10

Quadratus lumborum (beneath thoracolumbar fascia) 11

Quadriceps 2

Tibialis anterior 4

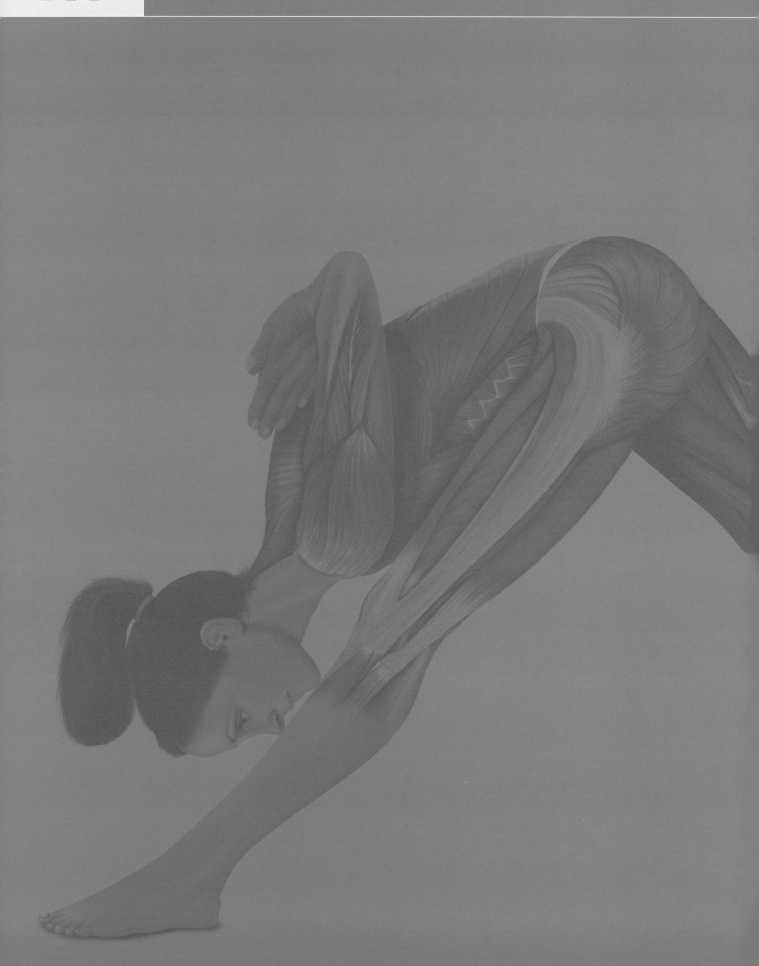

Standing Forward Bends

Forward bends, when practiced from a standing position, are effective in stretching the whole spine, especially the lower back area. They also stretch the back of the hips and legs and so are especially beneficial for those who partake in sports that tighten these areas, such as running and cycling. They also help to improve posture by lengthening the muscles that surround the spine and back of the pelvis.

On a mental level, forward bends have a calming effect and encourage inward reflection, leading to a decrease in anxiety and an increase in mental well-being.

Standing Forward Bend

Uttanasana

The Standing Forward Bend is a calming, therapeutic forward bend that can be performed by both beginners and people with advanced yoga experience, either as a stand-alone pose or as part of a sequence. The forward bend occurs as the hip flexors shorten and the gluteal muscles and hamstrings lengthen, allowing for the upper body to hinge forward. As the upper body moves toward the lower body, the crown of the head moves toward the ground, and the back and neck muscles relax as the spine lengthens, helping to minimize lower back pain. With the head in this position, the brain is calmed and the heart rate automatically slows down, which has a therapeutic effect on the nervous system. The arms are relaxed and the hands press lightly onto the ground, which encourages the spine to extend farther. The upper back muscles, mainly the trapezius, gently contract to draw the shoulders away from the head. The legs are straight with the body's weight distributed evenly through the feet. The calf muscles can be stretched farther by keeping the heels on the floor and transferring the weight slightly into the balls of the feet.

Level

Intermediate

Benefits

Standing Forward Bend is a calming asana that stretches the lower back and hamstrings and improves the function of the digestive system.

It can relieve pain in the lower back and is known for reducing stress, headaches, and fatigue.

Caution

People with low blood pressure, hamstring, or lower back injuries should be cautious when practicing this asana.

⊕ Modifications and props

Place the feet hips' width apart to make balancing easier.

To relieve pressure in the lower back, or if the hamstrings are injured, bend the knees.

If the hands do not reach the ground, place them on yoga bricks.

For excessive tension in the neck, also place a yoga brick under the crown of the head to provide additional support.

Try to

To lengthen from the lumbar spine, try to tilt the pelvis forward so the coccyx draws upward.

Relax the upper body, especially the neck, and let it lengthen toward the ground.

Maintain even weight distribution through the feet to avoid stress on the knees and lower back.

Try not to

Avoid sinking the body's weight back into the heels.

Try not to let the shoulders lift up around the head, because this will create tension around the neck. Lift them away from the head instead.

How to do it

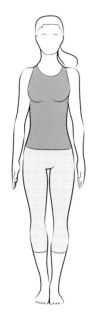

⊗ **Step 1**

Begin in Mountain Pose (page 54).

Step 2 ⊚

Make sure that the body's weight is distributed evenly through the feet and place the hands on the hips. Inhale and stretch the spine upward, so a sense of length is created around the lower back and the crown of the head feels as though it is being drawn gently upward.

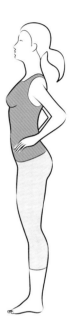

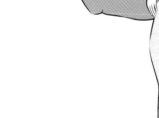

⊚ **Step 3**

Keeping the spine straight and the hands on the hips, breathe out deeply while extending the spine forward from the waist, moving the upper body toward the legs. The pelvis should be tilting forward with the spine elongating. Keep the legs straight and the toes relaxed, and maintain the weight evenly through the soles of the feet.

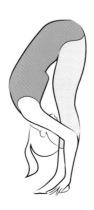

⊗ **Step 4**

Breathe steadily, and with the upper body pressing lightly on the front of the legs, rest the hands on the ground at each side of the feet. The fingers should be pointing forward and the elbows pointing backward. Press lightly into the hands to lengthen the spine. Now relax the neck completely and gently lift the shoulders away from the head to create a sense of space around the neck.

Standing Forward Bend

Uttanasana

The forward tilt of the pelvis in Standing Forward Bend occurs when the hip flexors, mainly the iliopsoas and rectus femoris, shorten via a concentric contraction. To let the hips tilt forward, the gluteus maximus and hamstrings have to lengthen eccentrically, and the gastrocnemius also lengthens when the legs straighten completely. The extensors of the spine, largely the erector spinae, relax and elongate eccentrically. The abdominal muscles isometrically contract to support the lumbar region while the trapezius muscles contract concentrically, moving the scapulae away from the head.

muscle activity

prime mover

1   Iliopsoas
2   Quadriceps
3   Rectus femoris
4   Trapezius

antagonist

5   Hamstrings
6   Erector spinae
7   Gluteus maximus
8   Gastrocnemius

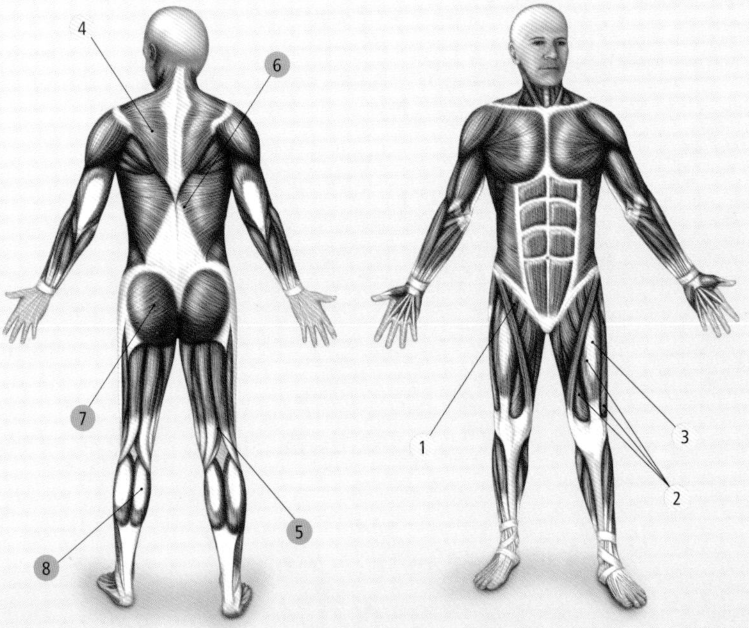

(6 beneath thoracolumbar fascia)

spine

The spine is in forward flexion, in a sagittal plane.
The pelvis is in an anterior tilt.

Anatomy of the pose

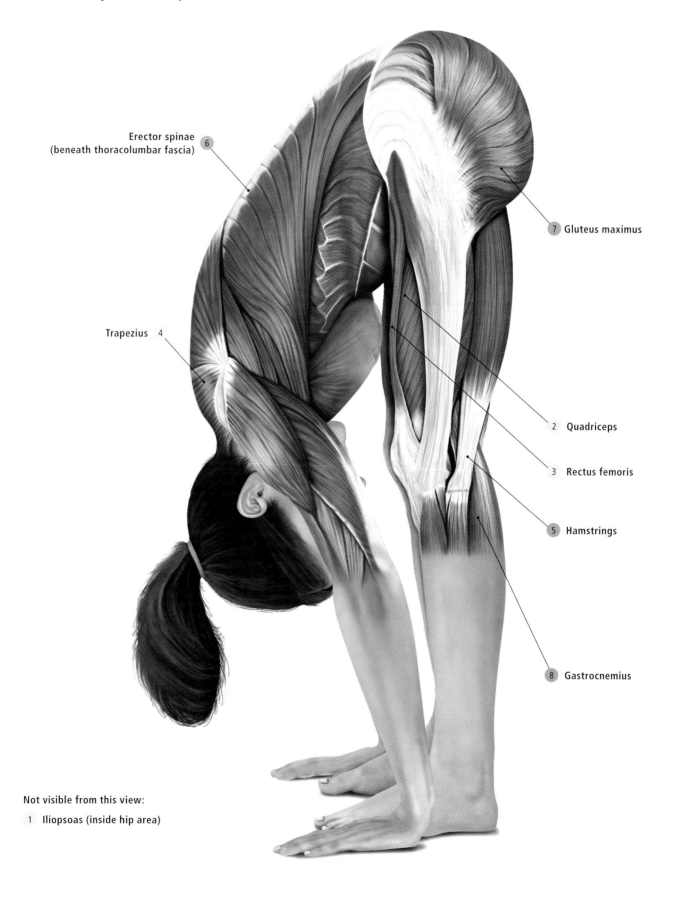

Erector spinae
(beneath thoracolumbar fascia) 6

7 Gluteus maximus

Trapezius 4

2 Quadriceps

3 Rectus femoris

5 Hamstrings

8 Gastrocnemius

Not visible from this view:

1 Iliopsoas (inside hip area)

Wide-Leg Forward Bend
Prasarita Padottanasana

The Wide-Leg Forward Bend is effective in improving the overall flexibility of the legs and lower back, which can, in turn, make other asanas, such as Triangle Pose and Extended Side-Angle Pose, more achievable. This asana is therapeutic for the spine, because the lengthening action of the upper body decompresses the vertebral disks and reduces tension by stretching the back muscles. This effect is initiated by a forward tilt of the pelvis, which occurs when the hamstrings and gluteus maximus muscles lengthen and the hip flexors shorten. The hips then tip forward, moving the spine into a forward-flexed position, lengthening all the lower back muscles. The wide-leg stance position also stretches the inner thighs, adductor muscles, and the outer ankles. The hands press into the ground with the elbows bent, which encourages the spine to lengthen farther, and the back muscles relax even more, moving the head closer to the ground. The shoulder blades move away from the head as the muscles of the upper back gently contract, which helps to relax the neck.

Level

Intermediate

Benefits

This asana can relieve lower back pain and greatly increases the flexibility of the hamstrings and adductor muscles.

Forward bends can also be effective at reducing fatigue and improving sleep patterns.

Caution

People with lower back injuries, or groin or hamstring strains should be cautious with when practicing this asana.

Deep forward bends can also affect blood pressure, so those with issues in this area should be careful to not overexert themselves.

⊕ Modifications and props

If the lower back is injured, bend the knees a little to reduce any pressure in the lumbar region.

For groin strains, make the stance shorter.

For low blood pressure, hold this asana for only up to ten breaths.

If it is not possible to reach the ground, place yoga bricks underneath the hands.

⊘ Try to

Lengthen the spine by drawing the tailbone upward and the crown of the head downward.

Create a strong foundation by pressing the feet firmly into the ground, so the feet and legs work more powerfully.

Place the hands so that they are in-line with the feet.

⊗ Try not to

Avoid taking the legs very wide so the asana is no longer stable.

Try not to drop the shoulders around the head. Instead, press firmly into the hands so the elbows move backward between the legs and the scapulae move down away from the head.

How to do it

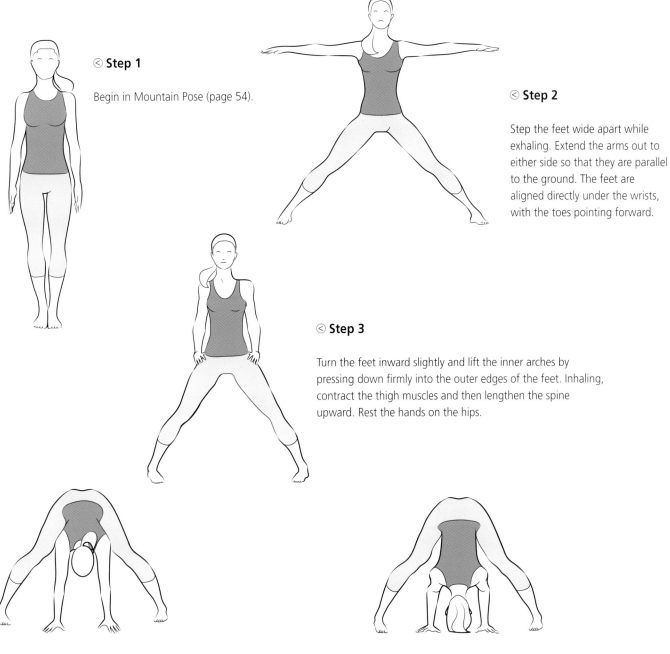

⊘ Step 1

Begin in Mountain Pose (page 54).

⊘ Step 2

Step the feet wide apart while exhaling. Extend the arms out to either side so that they are parallel to the ground. The feet are aligned directly under the wrists, with the toes pointing forward.

⊘ Step 3

Turn the feet inward slightly and lift the inner arches by pressing down firmly into the outer edges of the feet. Inhaling, contract the thigh muscles and then lengthen the spine upward. Rest the hands on the hips.

⋀ Step 4

Exhale slowly as the upper body folds forward from the hips, keeping the spine straight and the shoulders drawing back, away from the head. Pause when the spine is parallel to the ground and place the hands on the floor, aligned directly underneath the shoulders, with the arms straight. Inhale and press the seat bones backward as the spine lengthens forward. Rest the gaze on the ground.

⋀ Step 5

Exhale and fold more deeply from the lower back, so the head moves toward the ground. Place the hands in-line with the feet. The elbows point back between the legs, with the forearms perpendicular to the floor and the upper arms parallel to the floor. The legs remain straight, the neck is now relaxed and the entire spine is lengthening.

Wide-Leg Forward Bend

Prasarita Padottanasana

In this pose, the gluteus minimus and medius muscles contract concentrically and the adductors eccentrically contract, separating the legs away from the medial line of the body and creating a wide stance. The outer edges of the feet then press down into the ground as the peroneus longus lengthens eccentrically and the inner arches of the feet lift a little; this lift is maintained by the tibialis posterior and anterior. The forward flexion of the spine is due to a concentric shortening of the Iliopsoas and rectus femoris hip flexor muscles, and an eccentric lengthening of the hamstrings, gluteus maximus, erector spinae, soleus, and gastrocnemius. The trapezius muscles contract concentrically to lift the scapulae away from the ears and the biceps brachii shorten to flex the elbow joints.

muscle activity

prime mover

1   Iliopsoas
2   Rectus femoris
3   Quadriceps
4   Trapezius
5   Peroneus longus
6   Gluteus medius and minimus

antagonist

7   Hamstrings
8   Erector spinae
9   Gluteus maximus
10 Gastrocnemius
11 Soleus
12 Adductors

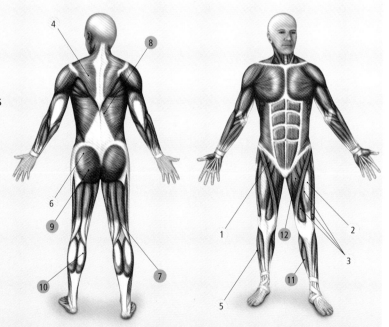

(6 beneath gluteus maximus; 8 beneath thoracolumbar fascia)

spine

The spine is in forward flexion in a sagittal plane, moving from a frontal plane axis.
The pelvis is in an anterior tilt.

Anatomy of the pose

Not visible from this view:

1 Iliopsoas (inside hip area, deep)
7 Hamstrings (rear of thigh)

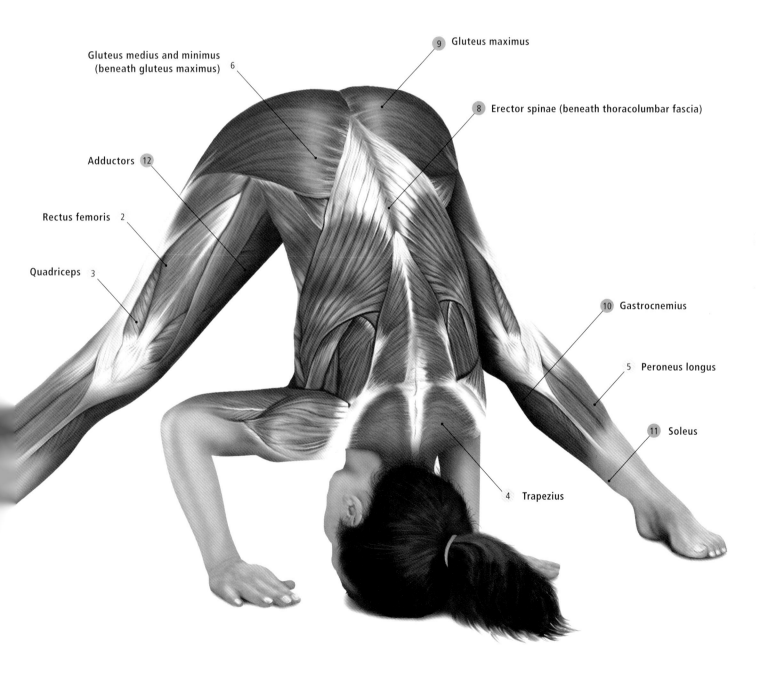

Gluteus medius and minimus
(beneath gluteus maximus) 6

9 Gluteus maximus

Adductors 12

8 Erector spinae (beneath thoracolumbar fascia)

Rectus femoris 2

Quadriceps 3

10 Gastrocnemius

5 Peroneus longus

11 Soleus

4 Trapezius

Intense Side Stretch

Parsvottanasana

Intense Side Stretch is a deep stretch for the hamstrings, calf muscles, back of the hips, and lower back. It aims to create space along the spine and through the upper body. The spine bends from the pelvis, which is tilting forward, and moves toward the right leg. This creates a strong stretch through the hamstrings and gluteal muscles, which lengthen, and a contraction through the hip flexors. The heels are aligned in a straight line, which means this posture requires a good balance and the person's complete focus. The small stabilizing muscles of the ankles have to contract to maintain this alignment of the ankle joints. The arms are in Reverse Prayer Position, with the hands behind the back, which helps to open and stretch the chest and front of the shoulders. By pressing the hands together in this way, the wrist flexors stretch and the upper back muscles contract and draw the shoulder blades toward one another, opening the shoulders farther.

Level

Intermediate

Benefits

This asana stretches the lower body, mainly the hamstrings and gluteal and calf muscles, and opens the chest and front of the shoulders.

It improves balance and mental focus and also stability of the ankle joints.

Caution

People with wrist, ankle, or lower back injuries should modify this asana.

Forward bends can affect low blood pressure, so again, caution should be taken when practicing this pose.

⊕ Modifications and props

If it is not possible to place the hands behind the back, fold the arms behind the back and hold each elbow instead, drawing the scapulae toward one another to keep the front of the shoulders open.

For lower back issues, bend the knee of the front leg a little.

For ankle injuries, position the feet diagonally to make balancing easier.

⊘ Try to

Before folding forward, align the right side of the pelvis with the left side, so it is in a neutral position, and stretch the spine upward.

Contract the thigh muscles and spread out the toes to improve balance.

⊗ Try not to

Try not to round the spine when folding forward; instead, focus on elongating the spine from the lower back to the neck.

Avoid the right hip moving forward and focus on moving it back, so it remains in-line with the left hip.

Do not lift the head when in the final phase of the asana. Let the neck relax, with the gaze resting on the middle of the lower leg.

How to do it

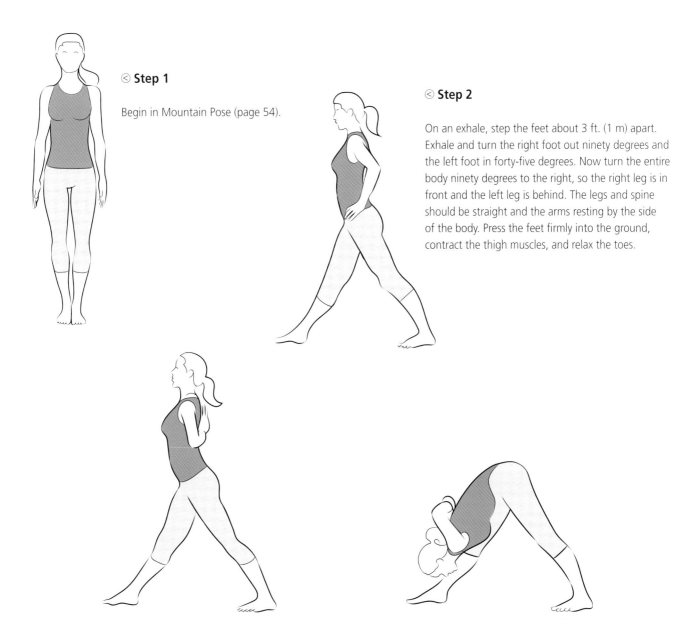

◉ **Step 1**

Begin in Mountain Pose (page 54).

◉ **Step 2**

On an exhale, step the feet about 3 ft. (1 m) apart. Exhale and turn the right foot out ninety degrees and the left foot in forty-five degrees. Now turn the entire body ninety degrees to the right, so the right leg is in front and the left leg is behind. The legs and spine should be straight and the arms resting by the side of the body. Press the feet firmly into the ground, contract the thigh muscles, and relax the toes.

◉ **Step 3**

Now begin to internally rotate the arms from the shoulder joints, so that the palms of the hands face backward. Bend the elbows and place the back of the hands onto the middle of the back while exhaling. Press the thumbs together and move the elbows backward to help stretch the chest area; this is known as Reverse Prayer Position. On an inhale, lift the sternum upward and lift the chin away from the chest to create a slight extension of the spine.

◉ **Step 4**

Exhale deeply and hinge forward by tilting the pelvis forward and extending from the lower back. Keep the legs straight as the upper body moves slowly toward the front leg, and keep pressing the hands together. Once the front of the rib cage is resting on the right leg, let the neck relax and bring the gaze toward the middle of the right lower leg. Continue to breathe deeply.

Intense Side Stretch

Parsvottanasana

For the Reverse Prayer Position of the hands used in this pose, the shoulder rotators inwardly rotate the humerus bones and the biceps brachii shorten, while the triceps lengthen to allow for flexion at the elbow. This allows for the hands to be positioned behind the middle spine with the wrists extended and the palms together. The anterior deltoids eccentrically stretch while the posterior deltoids and trapezius assist in drawing the scapulae together, creating a stretch across the chest. The quadriceps are concentrically contracted, extending the knee joints, while the sartorius hip flexor muscle, and other hip external rotators, externally rotates the left leg. The forward flexion of the spine is caused initially by a concentric shortening of the iliopsoas, resulting in a forward tilt of the pelvis. The erector spinae, quadratus lumborum, and hamstrings lengthen eccentrically to allow for this movement.

muscle activity

prime mover

1 Iliopsoas
2 Sartorius
3 Quadriceps
4 Deltoids
5 Biceps brachii
6 Trapezius
7 Wrist extensors

antagonist

8 Erector spinae
9 Quadratus lumborum
10 Hamstrings
11 Pectoralis major and minor
12 Triceps

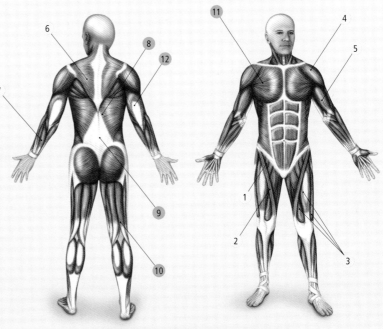

(8 and 9 beneath thoracolumbar fascia)

spine

The spine moves in a sagittal plane from a frontal axis and is in forward flexion.
The pelvis is in an anterior tilt.

Anatomy of the pose

Not visible from this view:

1 Iliopsoas (inside hip area, deep)

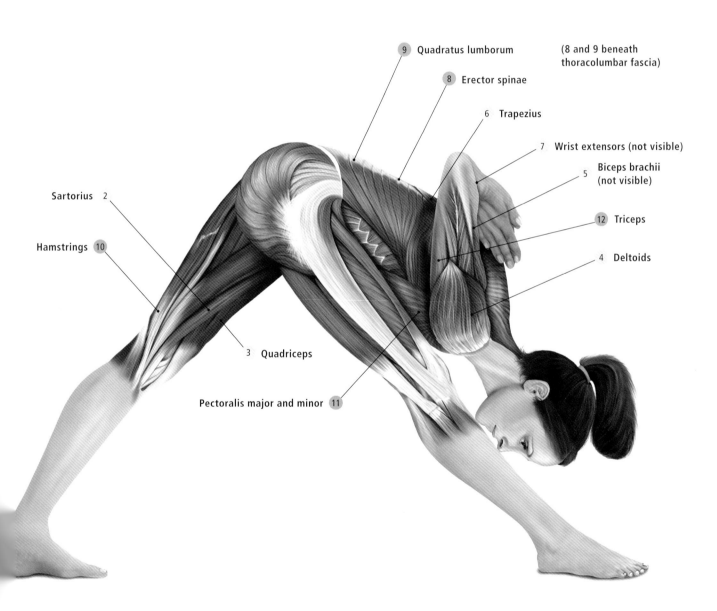

9 Quadratus lumborum

(8 and 9 beneath thoracolumbar fascia)

8 Erector spinae

6 Trapezius

7 Wrist extensors (not visible)

5 Biceps brachii (not visible)

Sartorius 2

12 Triceps

Hamstrings 10

4 Deltoids

3 Quadriceps

Pectoralis major and minor 11

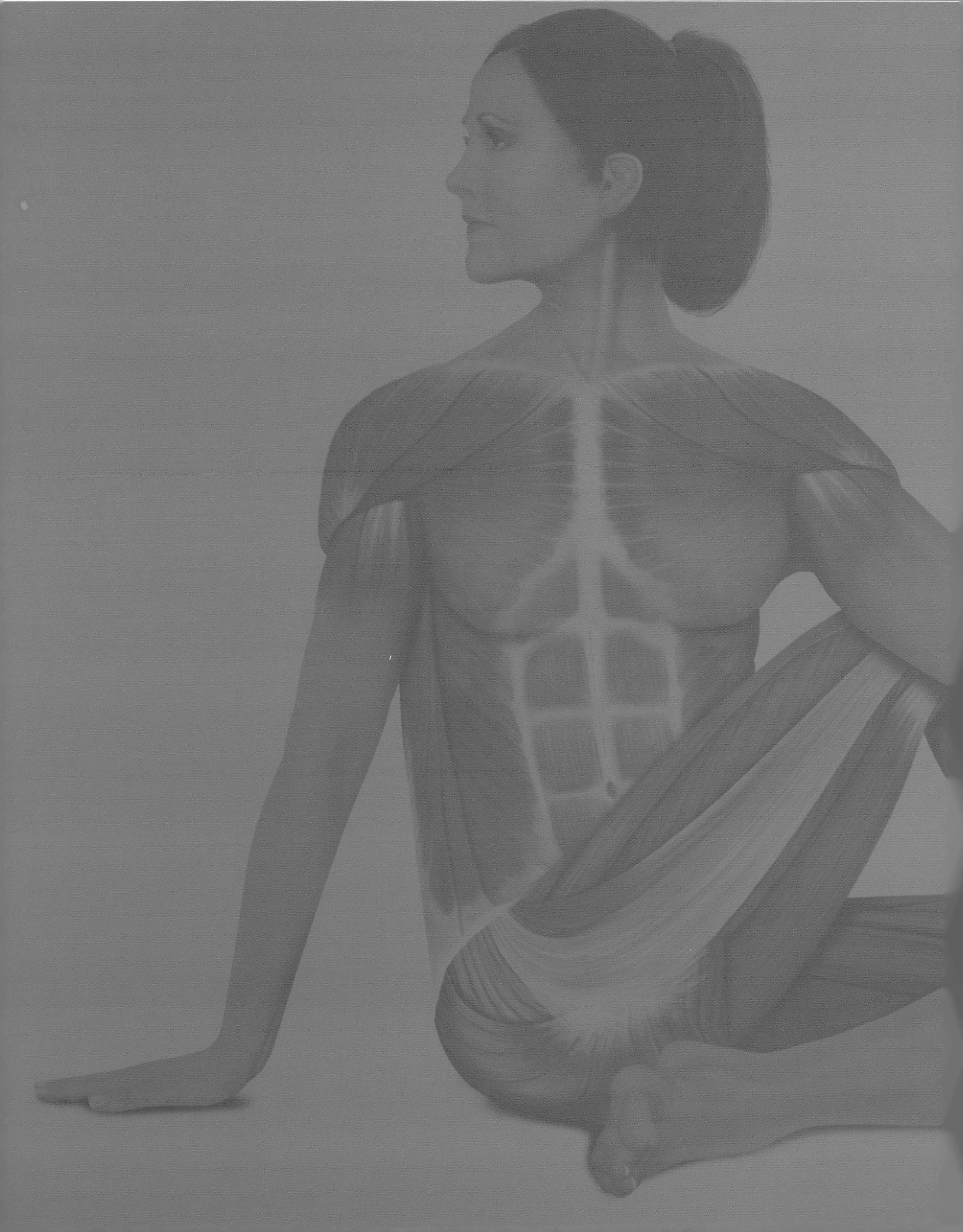

Seated Poses

Seated yoga asanas may involve twists, forward bends, or simply sitting with the spine straight and are mainly practiced after a standing yoga sequence. They are generally less demanding than standing asanas, because fewer muscle groups are utilized, but they can be more challenging mentally for some people, because the body needs to remain still. In this way, seated yoga postures can be used for quiet contemplation and are also useful for some people with limited mobility. Some seated yoga asanas, in which the spine remains straight, are also useful when practicing pranayama, because the lungs are not compressed in any way.

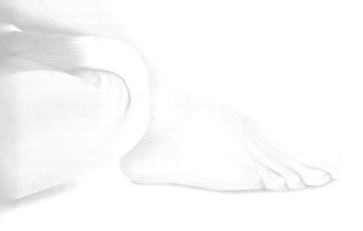

Seated Forward Bend

Paschimottanasana

The Seated Forward Bend is an effective stretch for the hamstrings, calf muscles, and lower back. The pelvis tilts forward and the spine extends forward, which encourages the body's weight to move onto the front part of the seat bones and then increases the stretch in the hamstrings and lower back. The legs are completely extended from the knee joint, with the quadriceps contracting and helping to press the legs together. The hands are positioned around the outer edges of the feet, helping to stretch the calf muscles farther. The position of the feet also helps to lengthen the Achilles tendon and the ligaments of the ankle joint. The shoulders draw down away from the head, which gives a sense of length in the upper back and neck. By stretching the spine and back of the legs like this, postural alignment is improved, because it becomes easier to straighten the spine when standing. By lowering the upper body and head, the heart rate is reduced, helping to calm the nervous system and, therefore, the mind.

Level

Beginner

Benefits

The Seated Forward Bend stretches the back of the legs and lumbar region and creates a sense of length through the entire body.

Because the abdomen rests on the thighs, this asana also helps to stimulate digestion.

Caution

If the lower back is injured, which includes injuries to the spinal disks, be careful when practicing this pose.

If the hamstrings or calf muscles are strained, the knees should be slightly bent.

Modifications and props

If it is not possible to straighten the spine, place a yoga block directly underneath the seat bones. This will encourage a more neutral alignment.

If the lower back is injured, bend the knees a little and place a rolled-up yoga mat behind the knees to support them.

If the feet cannot be reached, a yoga strap can be used.

⊘ Try to

Maintain length through the spine and draw the shoulders down, away from the head, so the neck also lengthens.

Maintain a sense of strength through the lower body by contracting the thigh muscles, pressing into the heels and keeping the toes pointing upward.

⊗ Try not to

Try not to round the spine and avoid lifting the shoulders toward the head. Instead, focus on elongating the spine from the lower back by tilting the pelvis forward.

Avoid pulling on the feet strongly, because this may cause strain.

Do not look directly forward, because this might strain the neck; instead, rest the gaze on the lower legs.

How to do it

Step 1 ⊙

Begin in Staff Pose (page 54).

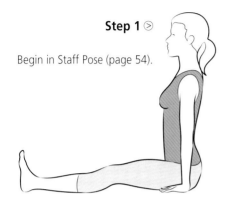

Step 2 ⊙

Inhale while extending the arms directly upward in-line with the ears. Keep the shoulders drawn down away from the head. Press into the heels and flex the feet, pointing the toes directly upward.

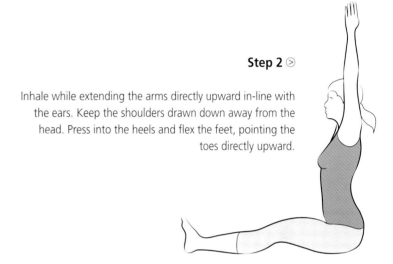

Step 3 ⊙

Keeping the arms in-line with the ears, begin to exhale and at the same time tilt the pelvis forward so the spine extends forward. Contract the abdominal muscles to support the lower back and maintain the strength through the legs.

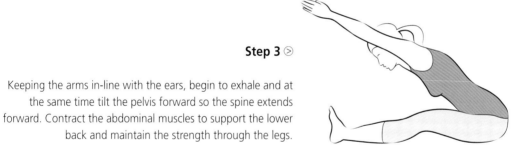

⊙ **Step 4**

Now lower the hands to the outside edges of the feet and slowly fold forward. On an exhale, bring the front of the upper body to rest on the legs. The elbows should point out on each side and the hands should gently pull on the outside edges of the feet to help lengthen the spine and the stretch through the back of the legs. Move the crown of the head toward the feet and relax the neck, resting the gaze on the lower legs. Continue to breathe deeply.

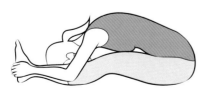

Seated Forward Bend

Paschimottanasana

In this pose, the quadriceps are concentrically contracting, while the hamstrings are eccentrically lengthening, resulting in full extension of the knee joints. The tibialis anterior are concentrically contracting, creating dorsiflexion of the ankle. This then eccentrically lengthens the hamstrings, soleus, and gastrocnemius, with the stretch increased farther when moving into the complete asana. The pelvis tilts forward when the iliopsoas shortens, creating a forward flexion at the lumbar spine. The gluteus maximus and erector spinae then lengthen eccentrically, letting the spine fold forward. The scapulae are drawn down away from the head when the trapezius and serratus anterior muscles contract concentrically.

prime mover

1 Iliopsoas
2 Quadriceps
3 Serratus anterior
4 Tibialis anterior
5 Trapezius

antagonist

6 Hamstrings
7 Erector spinae
8 Gluteus maximus
9 Soleus and gastrocnemius

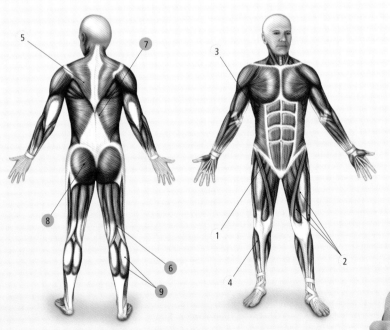

(7 beneath thoracolumbar fascia)

The spine moves in a sagittal plane from a frontal axis and is in forward flexion.
The pelvis is in an anterior tilt.

Anatomy of the pose

Not visible from this view:

1 Iliopsoas (inside hip area, deep)
4 Tibialis anterior (lower leg)
9 Soleus and gastrocnemius (lower leg)

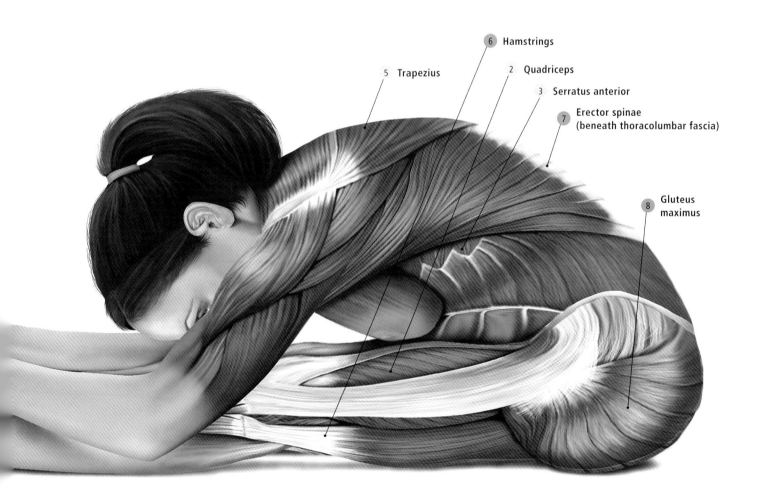

6 Hamstrings

5 Trapezius

2 Quadriceps

3 Serratus anterior

7 Erector spinae
(beneath thoracolumbar fascia)

8 Gluteus
maximus

Boat Pose

Navasana

Boat Pose is an intense asana that requires considerable strength of the abdominal, lower back, and leg muscles. To hold the spine in position, the abdominal and lower back muscles contract, supporting the lumbar region. The legs are completely extended and raised from the ground by a strong contraction of the iliopsoas, quadriceps, and hip flexors. The triceps muscles shorten to straighten the arms and hold them parallel to the floor, and the shoulder blades are drawn together and down, away from the ears. This action helps the sternum lift upward slightly, encouraging a sense of lift and length from the lower back, and making sure the core muscles work even harder. Regular practice of Boat Pose helps overall strength and endurance, especially of the core muscles. This, in turn, helps improve the performance of other asanas that require a good deal of core stability, such as Headstand Pose. Because the iliopsoas and hip flexors shorten in Boat Pose, follow this asana with a hip-opening pose, such as Cobbler's Pose or Pigeon Pose, to stretch these muscles.

Level

Intermediate

Benefits

Boat Pose significantly increases the strength of the lower back and abdominal area. The muscles that support the pelvis—the iliopsoas—also strengthen, because they help to move the legs closer to the torso. Mental focus is also improved.

Caution

Boat Pose works the lower back powerfully, so people with lower back injuries should modify this asana. Those with hernias should not practice Boat Pose.

⊕ **Modifications and props**

To minimize pressure on the lower back, bend the knees so the lower legs are level to the floor. For additional support, hold the backs of the thighs. This will make it easier to lift the sternum and stop the spine from rounding.

 Try to

Contract the abdominal muscles powerfully to support the lower back area. Aim to lift the sternum upward and move the shoulder blades toward one another, so the lower back does not curve and excessive pressure is not put on the lumbar spine.

Try to press the legs together firmly, so all the muscles of the legs are working.

 Try not to

Try not to round the spine, because this may put pressure on the lower back.

Avoid lowering the legs to a point where there is strain on the hip flexors. Instead, focus on maintaining the neutral alignment of the spine and keep the feet in-line with the gaze.

How to do it

Step 1 ⊙

Begin in Staff Pose (page 54).

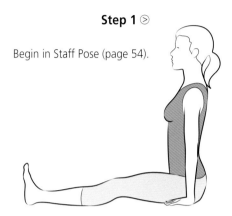

Step 2 ⊙

Bend the legs so that the feet are flat to the floor and there is about 20 in. (50 cm) between the seat bones and the heels. Place the hands lightly around the back of the thighs. Transfer the body's weight toward the back of the pelvis and lean the spine back slightly, keeping it in a straight line. Contract the abdominal muscles so the spine is supported. Breathe evenly throughout.

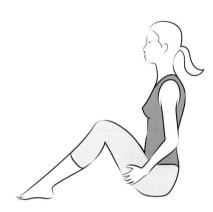

⊙ **Step 3**

Inhale while lifting the feet so that the lower legs are parallel to the ground. Press the legs together and extend the arms forward so that they are also parallel to the ground. The palms should be facing toward one another. Continue to breathe steadily and move the shoulder blades toward one another, so the chest lifts a little. The chin should be level to the floor.

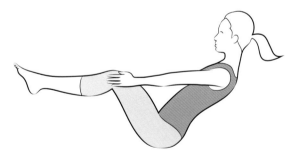

Step 4 ⊙

Now, on an exhale, completely extend the legs, contracting the muscles of the legs strongly and pressing the legs together more firmly. Keep the chest lifted and the arms level with the ground. The abdominal muscles will need to work more powerfully now and should be drawn in toward the spine. Breathe steadily throughout.

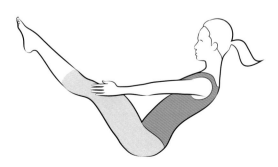

Boat Pose

Navasana

In Boat Pose, the hip flexors, mainly the iliopsoas, are concentrically shortened, moving the legs toward the torso and the hips into a partly flexed position. The pelvis is tilted back so the majority of the body's weight is on the coccyx and ischium bones. The spine is in a slightly extended position and angled back, so that the spine and legs make a "V" shape.

To support the position of the spine, the rectus and transversus abdominis works powerfully as fixators, as does the erector spinae and latissimus dorsi. The quadriceps and soleus are concentrically contracting to completely extend the legs and ankles, as are the triceps to extend the arms from the elbow joints. The anterior deltoids fixate the arms in place and the posterior deltoids hold the scapulae in place.

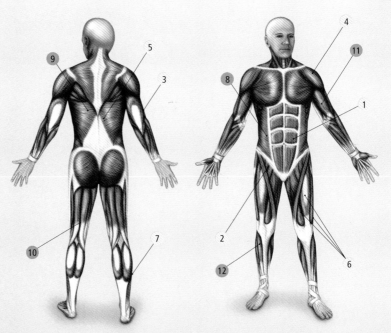

prime mover

1	Rectus abdominis
2	Iliopsoas
3	Triceps
4	Deltoids
5	Erector spinae
6	Quadriceps
7	Soleus

antagonist

8	Transversus abdominis
9	Latissimus dorsi
10	Hamstrings
11	Biceps brachii
12	Tibialis anterior

(5 beneath thoracolumbar fascia)

The spine is in a neutral position and moves on a sagittal plane from a frontal axis.
The pelvis is in an anterior tilt position.

Anatomy of the pose

Not visible from this view:

2   Iliopsoas (inside hip area, deep)

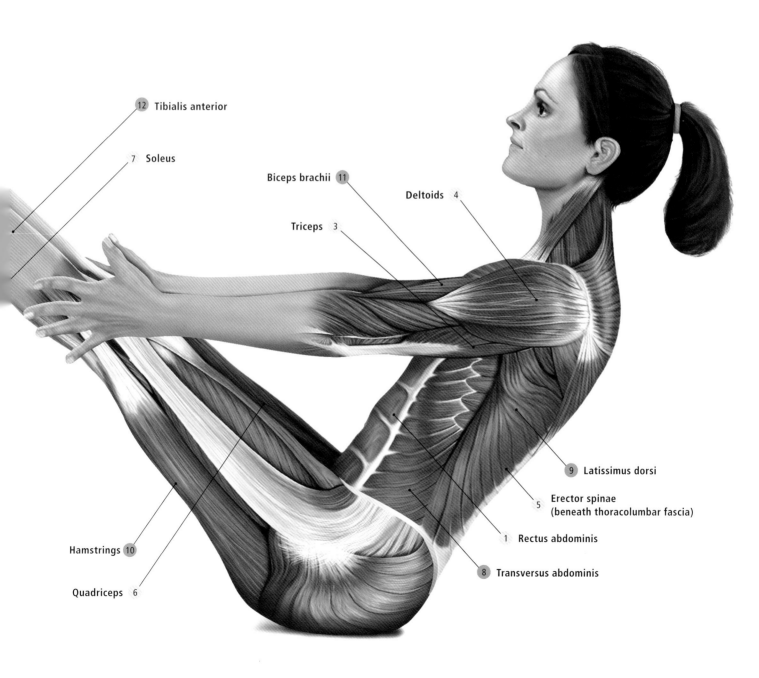

12 Tibialis anterior

7   Soleus

Biceps brachii 11

Deltoids 4

Triceps 3

9   Latissimus dorsi

5   Erector spinae
(beneath thoracolumbar fascia)

1   Rectus abdominis

8   Transversus abdominis

Hamstrings 10

Quadriceps 6

Half Lord of the Fishes Pose
Ardha Matsyendrasana

Half Lord of the Fishes is a therapeutic spinal twist that increases the flexibility of the spine. The rotating action stretches the upper body on one side and compresses the other. On the compressed side, the internal organs are gently massaged, which is thought to have a detoxifying effect, especially on the digestive system.

The oblique abdominal muscles stretch on one side and lengthen on the other, while both sides of the back stretch and lengthen. The right arm is extended and supports the torso, while the left arm acts as a lever against the right leg to increase the rotation of the spine. The legs are bent, with the right foot pressing down into the ground, which encourages the spine to extend upward, and the left leg is relaxed on the floor. This position of the legs helps to stretch the hips and gluteal muscles, which, in turn, can help alleviate lower backache. The overall effect of this asana is a gentle stretch into the hips and shoulders and a strong stretch of the back muscles.

Level

Intermediate

Benefits

This asana increases the spine's flexibility by stretching the back muscles and connective tissues of the rib cage. It also stretches the hips.

The twisting action of the upper body gently stimulates the internal organs, which improves their general functioning.

Caution

This twisting action is not appropriate for spinal disk injuries or injuries to the neck.

Those with conditions affecting the knee joint may need to modify the position of the legs.

⊕ Modifications and props

If the spine is rounded, place a yoga block underneath the hips. This will help to bring the pelvis and lower back into a more neutral alignment.

If the knees are injured, keep the left leg straight and move the right foot away from the hips a little.

⊘ Try to

Elongate the spine by extending it upward before twisting. Press the right foot into the ground to assist with this action.

For a deeper twist, press the left arm against the right outer thigh more firmly, but not to the point of overexertion.

⊗ Try not to

Avoid rounding the spine, because this will put undue pressure on the spinal disks.

Don't twist the neck too far; instead, turn the head gently toward the right shoulder.

Avoid pressing the left arm too strongly against the right thigh.

How to do it

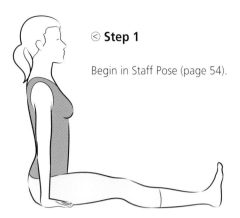

⊘ Step 1

Begin in Staff Pose (page 54).

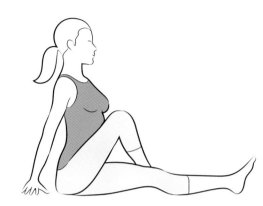

⊘ Step 2

Bend the right knee and place the right foot on the ground next to the outer left hip, so the right leg is positioned over the left thigh. The sole of the right foot should be on the ground with the toes pointing forward. The spine remains straight. Make sure breathing is slow and even.

Step 3 ⊗

Now bend the left leg and place the left foot next to the right outer hip. The left leg should be relaxed with the entire outer ankle, foot, and right leg resting on the ground. Flex the left foot by moving the left toes toward the left shin, creating flexion in the ankle joint. Press the right foot into the ground to create more lift through the upper body.

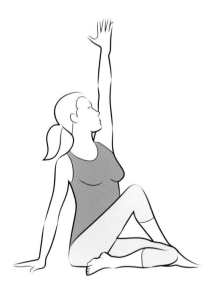

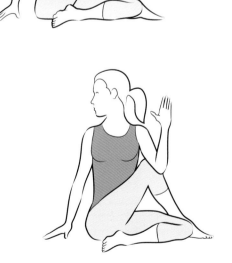

⌃ Step 4

Place the right hand on the ground behind the back, in-line with the coccyx, and extend the left arm directly upward on an inhale. Feel the lift and length through the entire spine as the upper body rotates toward the right on an exhale. The left shoulder should be moving forward and the right shoulder backward.

⌃ Step 5

On an exhale, bend the left elbow and place it firmly against the outer right thigh. The fingers and thumb of the left hand should be pointing directly up and the left arm pressing firmly against the outer right thigh to increase the rotation of the spine. The chin should be parallel to the ground and the gaze over the right shoulder. Breathe steadily.

Half Lord of the Fishes Pose

Ardha Matsyendrasana

In this sitting twist, the quadriceps stretch eccentrically to allow for the flexion at the knee joints, which is instigated by the hamstrings contracting concentrically. The iliopsoas on the right side contract concentrically to flex and adduct the right thigh and bring it in toward the upper body. The left side of the hip is externally rotated and iliopsoas lengthens eccentrically to abduct the leg away from the upper body, so it can rest on the ground. The oblique muscles work on each side of the torso to create the rotation of the thoracic spine and rib cage, with the right side obliques shortening concentrically and the left side obliques lengthening eccentrically. The latissimus dorsi also lengthens and shortens in the same way and the rectus abdominis works isometrically to support the upper body. The left arm is flexed at the elbow due to the concentric shortening of the biceps brachii, and the right arm is externally rotated and completely extended at the elbow due to the triceps also shortening concentrically.

muscle activity

prime mover

1 Internal and external obliques
2 Hamstrings
3 Latissimus dorsi
4 Iliopsoas

antagonist

5 Quadriceps
6 Rectus abdominis
7 Erector spinae
8 Semispinalis thoracis
9 Gluteus maximus

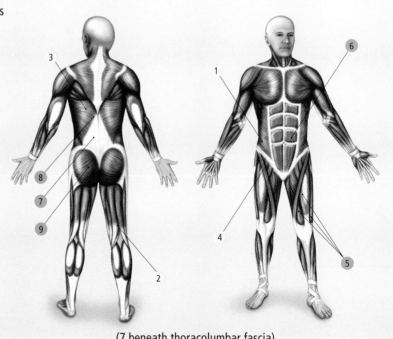

(7 beneath thoracolumbar fascia)

spine

The spine is in rotation in a neutral position and is not moving within a plane.
The pelvis is also in a neutral position, because it is not tilted.

Anatomy of the pose

Not visible from this view:

4 Iliopsoas (inside hip area, deep)
7 Erector spinae
8 Semispinalis thoracis

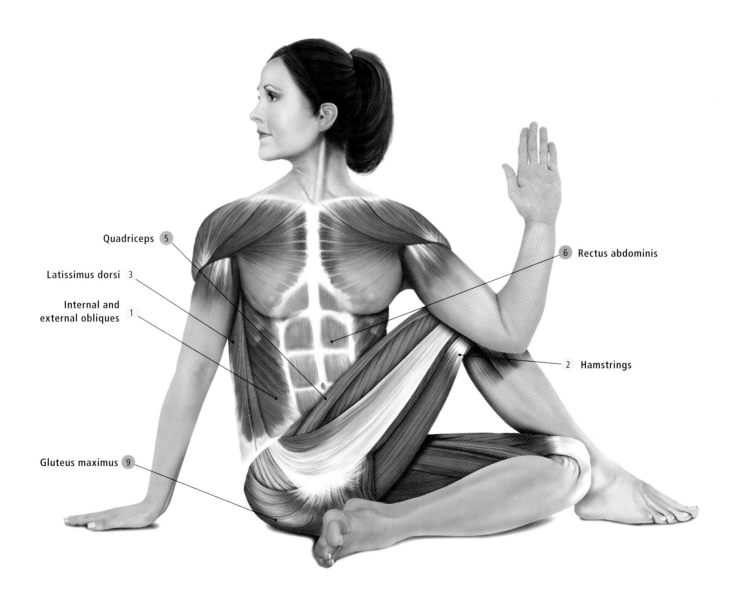

Quadriceps 5

Latissimus dorsi 3

Internal and
external obliques 1

Gluteus maximus 9

6 Rectus abdominis

2 Hamstrings

Cobbler's Pose

Baddha Konasana

Cobbler's Pose is a hip-opening asana that improves the flexibility of the hips and stretches the lower back. It aims to stretch the inner thigh muscles and groin, and it is effective for preparing the hips for other hip-opening asanas, such as Pigeon Pose and Dancer's Pose.

The smaller gluteal muscles around the outer hips shorten to move the thighbones out to each side, which then let the soles of the feet come together. This action not only stretches the ankles but also lengthens the inner thigh muscles, and it stretches the connective tissue around the knee joints, too. The pelvis at this point is in a neutral position. To flex the spine forward over the ankles and feet, the spine moves into a forward-tilt position. This greatly intensifies the stretch in the inner thigh and groin, and the lower back and back of the gluteal muscles are also stretched. The hands are placed around the feet and the arms are bent with the elbows resting on the inner legs, which helps to stretch the inner thighs and hips farther.

Level

Intermediate

Benefits

The Cobbler's Pose opens the hips and stretches the inner thighs. It can help to alleviate lower backache and has been known to alleviate sciatica.

Caution

For those with either groin or knee injuries, be careful when practicing Cobbler's Pose.

For people with lower back injuries, such as a herniated vertebral disk, the forward bend part of this asana should not be practiced.

Modifications and props

If the hips are inflexible, remain in an upright position and let the legs relax without bending forward.

To take pressure off the knees, move the feet farther away from the pelvis.

If the pelvis is tilting backward, place a yoga block underneath the pelvis to bring it into a neutral alignment.

⊘ Try to

Focus on lifting the spine upward and let the legs relax toward the ground slowly, so the front of the hips open gradually.

When folding the upper body forward, the spine should remain elongated.

The elbows can press onto the inner thighs to increase the stretch of the hips, but avoid this adjustment if the hips are inflexible.

⊗ Try not to

Try not to round the spine. Instead, lengthen the spine upward and lift the sternum a little, and maintain the length through the upper body when folding forward.

To avoid tension in the shoulders and neck area, keep the shoulders down, away from the head.

How to do it

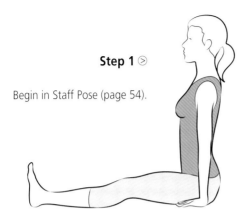

Step 1 ⊚

Begin in Staff Pose (page 54).

Step 2 ⊚

Bend the knees until the heels are a couple of inches away from the pelvis and bring the soles of the feet together. Now exhale while letting the legs drop to each side, moving them toward the ground. Move the heels as close to the pelvis as you can without feeling pressure in the knees, and place the hands around the feet with the fingers interlaced. The spine should be upright and straight. Now inhale and at the same time lift the sternum a little, drawing the shoulders down away from the head. Press the feet together and let the legs move closer to the ground by relaxing the hips.

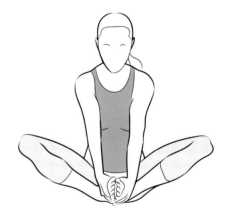

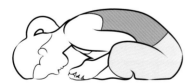

⊚ **Step 3**

Now exhale slowly while the pelvis tilts forward and the upper body extends forward. The chest should be moving toward the feet with the stretch of the inner thighs increasing. The elbows should be resting on the inner legs. Keep breathing deeply as the head and neck relax, and rest the gaze on the toes.

Cobbler's Pose

Baddha Konasana

The quadriceps are eccentrically lengthened and the hamstrings are concentrically contracted, completely flexing the knees. The piriformis, sartorius, and gluteus medius and minimus all work in unison and contract concentrically to externally rotate the femurs, allowing for the soles of the feet to press together and the legs to rest on the floor. In this position, the adductors stretch eccentrically. The pelvis is in an anterior tilt position, and quadratus lumborum and erector spinae stretch eccentrically to let the spine flex forward over the ankles and feet. The trapezius muscles move the scapulae away from the head and the biceps brachii shorten concentrically to flex the elbows.

muscle activity

prime mover

1 Gluteus medius and minimus
2 Sartorius
3 Trapezius
4 Piriformis
5 Hamstrings
6 Biceps brachii

antagonist

7 Adductors
8 Erector spinae
9 Quadratus lumborum

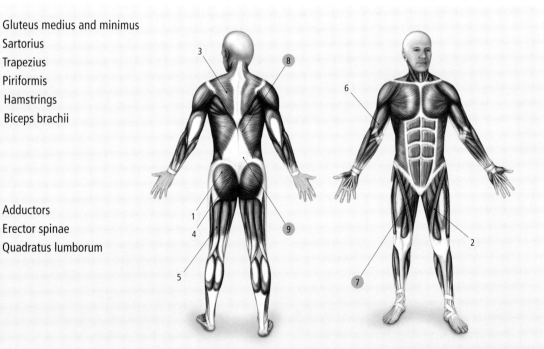

(1 and 4 beneath gluteus maximus; 8 and 9 beneath thoracolumbar fascia)

spine

The spine moves in a sagittal plane from a frontal axis and is in forward flexion.
The pelvis is in an anterior tilt position.

Anatomy of the pose

Not visible from this view:

1 Gluteus medius and minimus (beneath gluteus maximus)
4 Piriformis (beneath gluteus maximus)
6 Biceps brachii
8 Erector spinae (on back)

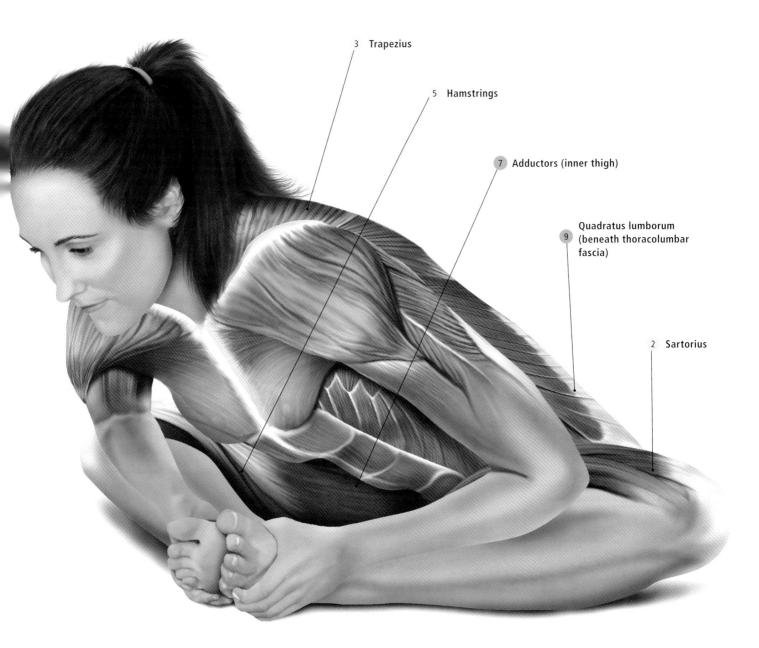

3 Trapezius

5 Hamstrings

7 Adductors (inner thigh)

9 Quadratus lumborum (beneath thoracolumbar fascia)

2 Sartorius

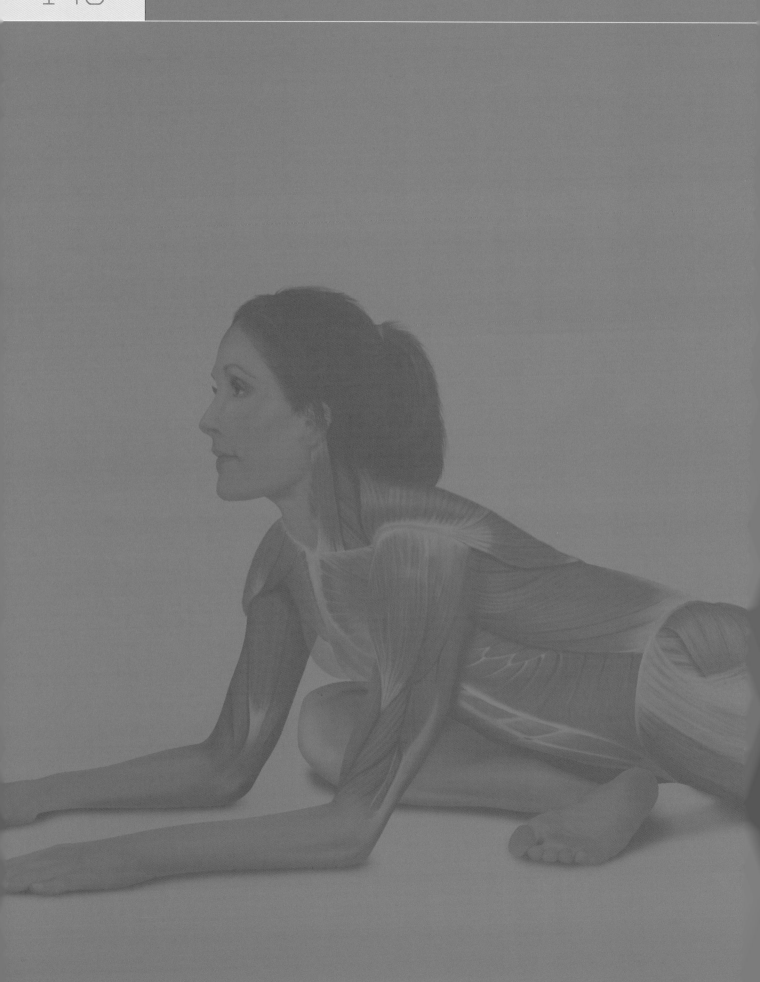

Backbend Poses

Backbending asanas extend the spine in the opposite direction to forward bends and are generally practiced toward the end of a hatha yoga session, when the body is warm and more flexible. They are effective in stretching the abdominal muscles and the hip flexors. In more advanced backbending asanas, such as Wheel Pose, the entire front of the body, including the shoulders and chest area, is also deeply stretched. This has a dramatic effect in improving overall flexibility.

Mentally, backbends are invigorating, leading to clarity of mind and increased energy levels within the body.

Cobra Pose

Bhujangasana

Cobra Pose is one of the gentler backbending asanas that strengthens the entire spine. The arms are in a flexed position and, as the hands press lightly into the ground and the chest lifts from the floor, the extensor muscles of the spine shorten and move into an extended position, which, in particular, increases the flexibility of the thoracic spine.

The muscles of the upper back, including the trapezius muscles, move the shoulder blades away from the head, allowing for the neck to elongate, so the entire upper body feels lengthened. The feet are stretched away from the body and press into the floor, which helps the thigh and gluteal muscles to contract. At the same time, the abdominal muscles lengthen and stretch, and the light pressure on the lower abdominal area has a therapeutic effect on the digestive system.

Level

Beginner

Benefits

Cobra Pose strengthens the legs and extensor muscles of the spine. It also stretches the abdominal and chest muscles.

Caution

People with vertebral disk or wrist injuries should be cautious when practicing Cobra Pose.

⊕ Modifications and props

In the case of back injuries, only lift the top part of the chest from the floor, so the extension of the spine is minimal. Also press into the hands more so the arms can provide more support to the spine.

For lower back injuries, separate the feet so they are hips' width apart.

For wrist injuries, avoid pressing firmly into the hands.

Try to

Maintain a sense of length through the spine and legs.

To create lift, use predominantly the muscles of the back instead of pressing into the hands and using only the arms.

Actively move the shoulders away from the ears to create space through the neck.

Try not to

Avoid lifting the chin beyond horizontal and compressing the back of the neck. Instead, aim to elongate the neck.

Try not to overwork the gluteal muscles by tensing them, because this may put undue tension on the lower back.

How to do it

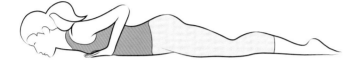

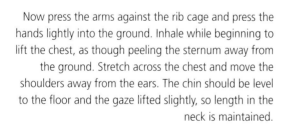

⊙ Step 1

From lying face down, place the hands on each side of the chest with the fingers and thumbs pointing forward. The legs should be pressed together and the feet stretched away. Press the tops of the feet into the ground and draw the heels toward one another. Contract the gluteal and thigh muscles. Maintain a steady breath throughout.

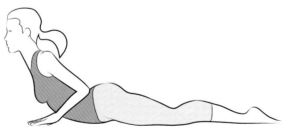

Step 2 ⊙

Now press the arms against the rib cage and press the hands lightly into the ground. Inhale while beginning to lift the chest, as though peeling the sternum away from the ground. Stretch across the chest and move the shoulders away from the ears. The chin should be level to the floor and the gaze lifted slightly, so length in the neck is maintained.

Cobra Pose

Bhujangasana

During Cobra Pose, the thoracic spine is in an extended position due to a concentric contraction of the erector spinae and latissimus dorsi muscle groups. The elbows are in a flexed position, with the triceps lengthening eccentrically and the biceps brachii shortening concentrically. The triceps then fixate the arms in place via an isometric contraction. The scapulae are moved down, away from the head and toward the spine, by the trapezius and rhomboid muscles. The hip and knee joints are completely extended, with the legs lengthening away from the torso and the tops of the feet pressed into the ground. The quadriceps contract concentrically and gluteus maximus contract isometrically, providing support for the sacroiliac and pelvic area. As the chest lifts, the pectoral and rectus abdominis muscles lengthen eccentrically, letting the spine extend and stretch away from the ground.

Anatomy of the pose

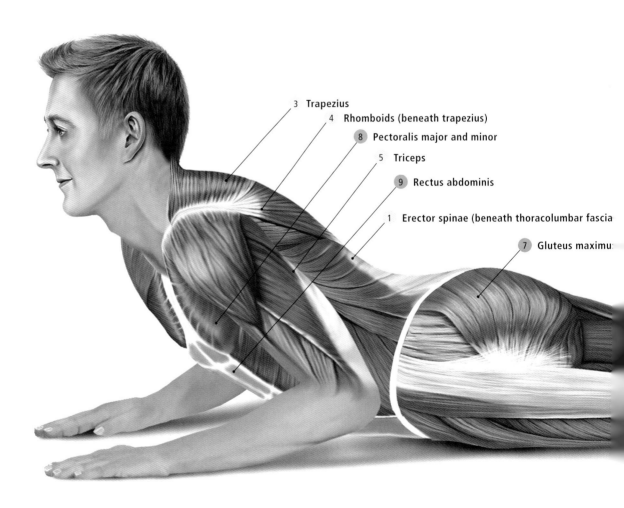

3 Trapezius
4 Rhomboids (beneath trapezius)
8 Pectoralis major and minor
5 Triceps
9 Rectus abdominis
1 Erector spinae (beneath thoracolumbar fascia
7 Gluteus maximu

muscle activity

prime mover

1 Erector spinae
2 Quadriceps
3 Trapezius
4 Rhomboids
5 Triceps

antagonist

6 Hamstrings
7 Gluteus maximus
8 Pectoralis major and minor
9 Rectus abdominis

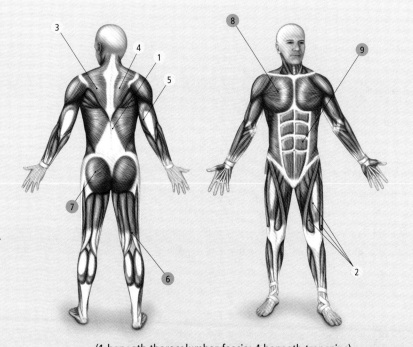

(1 beneath thoracolumbar fascia; 4 beneath trapezius)

spine

The spine is in an extended position and moves in a sagittal plane from a frontal axis.
The pelvis is in a neutral position.

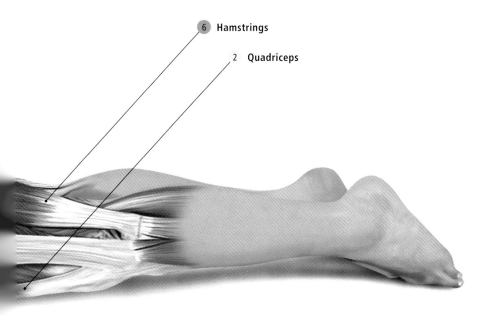

6 Hamstrings

2 Quadriceps

Upward-Facing Dog Pose
Urdhva Mukha Svanasana

This asana involves a backbending position and demands considerable strength from the arms and legs. The spine is in an extended position, which lengthens the muscles at the front on the body, in particular, the hip flexors and abdominal muscles. The legs are stretched back, with the feet hips' width apart, and the thighs and gluteal muscles work hard to support the lower back. The abdominal muscles, although stretched, also contract to support the lower back. The arms are extended, with the triceps contracting powerfully and helping to lift the upper body. The chest and front of the shoulders stretch while the muscles of the upper back work to move the shoulder blades downward. This action opens the whole of the front upper body, which, in turn, improves postural alignment. The chin is a little above parallel to the ground with the gaze lifted. This helps encourages a lifting action through the crown.

Level

Intermediate

Benefits

This asana improves posture by stretching the chest, shoulders, abdomen, and the front of the hips.

It increases the flexibility of the entire spine and energizes the body, relieving fatigue.

Caution

Those with back injuries should use caution when practicing this asana.

For conditions like herniated disks or wrist injuries, Upward-Facing Dog Pose should not be practiced. Cobra Pose is more appropriate.

⊕ Modifications and props

If it is too challenging to maintain the lift of the hips and legs off the floor, position a rolled-up blanket underneath the tops of the thighs. This will give the lower back more support.

⊘ Try to

Really lengthen through the entire spine and aim to create space within the upper body.

Press the feet firmly into the ground so the legs work powerfully. This will help to avoid pressure in the lower back.

To avoid undue tension in the neck area, try to move the shoulders away from the head and work the upper back to draw the shoulder blades downward.

⊗ Try not to

Avoid "hanging" from the shoulders. Instead, make sure the arms are working powerfully and the upper body is open.

Try not to relax the legs and instead keep the leg and gluteal muscles strong to support the spine.

Avoid taking the feet wider than hips' width apart, because this can put stress on the lower back area.

How to do it

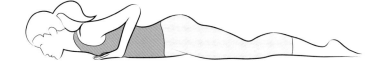

⊗ Step 1

Lie face down on the ground and stretch the legs straight back with the tops of the feet resting on the ground. Make sure the breath is even and that the feet are no more than hips' width apart. Now bend the elbows and place the palms of the hands on the ground on each side of the upper body, so they align about halfway down the rib cage. The forearms should be almost perpendicular to the ground. Spread the fingers and thumbs so the hands feel stretched.

⊗ Step 2

Inhale deeply and on the next exhale, press the hands firmly onto the ground, and begin to straighten the arms while simultaneously lifting the torso directly upward, until the legs and front of the hips also lift a few inches off the ground. The tops of the feet should remain on the ground. Stretch all the way to the toes and firm the legs so the gluteal muscles also contract.

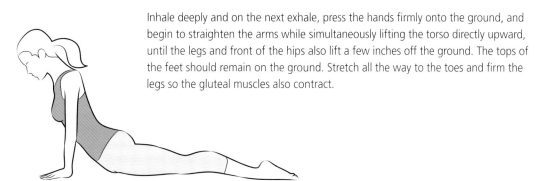

Step 3 ⊗

Breathing steadily, focus now on pressing the chest forward a little and drawing the shoulders down until the chest feels more open. As the front of the shoulders stretch, the inner elbows should face forward. Lift the chin slightly higher than parallel to the ground, maintaining the length through the neck and lifting the gaze upward at the same time.

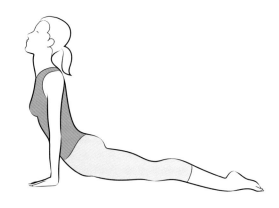

Upward-Facing Dog Pose

Urdhva Mukha Svanasana

In Upward-Facing Dog Pose, the triceps are in a concentric contraction and the biceps brachii are lengthened, completely extending the elbows and straightening the arms. Because the hands are directly underneath the shoulders, the entire spine then moves into an extended position, with a concentric contraction of the erector spinae and latissimus dorsi muscles. The rectus and transversus abdominis muscles eccentrically contract as the spine extends, and the anterior shoulders and inner elbows externally rotate, while the trapezius moves the scapulae downward, resulting in the pectoral muscles eccentrically lengthening. The quadriceps are concentrically contracted, extending the knees and straightening the legs. The hamstrings support this action by contracting isometrically, as do the gluteus maximus muscles. This supports the lumbar spine and sacroiliac area.

Anatomy of the pose

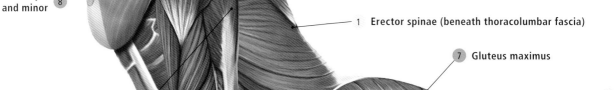

Deltoids 5

3 Trapezius

Pectoralis major and minor 8

1 Erector spinae (beneath thoracolumbar fascia)

7 Gluteus maximus

2 Quadriceps

Triceps 4

6 Hamstrings

Rectus abdominis 9

prime mover

1 Erector spinae
2 Quadriceps
3 Trapezius
4 Triceps
5 Deltoids

antagonist

6 Hamstrings
7 Gluteus maximus
8 Pectoralis major and minor
9 Rectus abdominis

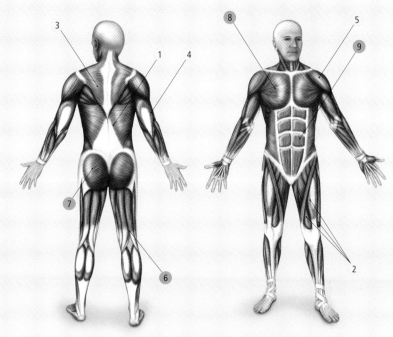

(1 beneath thoracolumbar fascia)

The spine is in an extended position and moves in a sagittal plane from a frontal axis.
The pelvis is in a posterior tilt position.

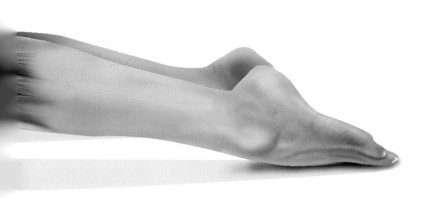

Pigeon Pose

Eka Pada Kapotasana

Pigeon Pose is a hip-opening asana that not only stretches the muscles of the pelvis but also prepares the hips for other asana, such as Dancer's Pose and Cobbler's Pose. The front leg is bent and the angle of the thigh and right knee stretches all the gluteal muscles of the right hip. This has a therapeutic effect on the lumbar region, and with regular practice, Pigeon Pose can ease recurrent lower back pain and sciatica, because it also stretches the muscles around the back of the pelvis.

The left leg is extended behind the body with the hip flexors stretching and lengthening. By extending the left foot away from the body, the ankle joint is stretched. The spine flexes forward over the right leg with the arms resting on the floor, which helps stretch the upper body. Opening the hips in this way increases the general mobility and flexibility of hip joints, ankles, and knees. Many athletes, such as runners and cyclists, find that Pigeon Pose can help maintain a healthy range of movement in the hips. Regular practice leads to a quicker recovery from training and a decreased risk of injury.

Level

Intermediate

Benefits

This asana stretches the muscles of the pelvic area, in particular, the gluteal muscles and hip flexors. This leads to improved posture and increases the ability to practice other yoga asanas that require a big range of movement through the hips without causing strain.

Caution

For injuries to the knee, such as damage to the tendons or ligaments, caution should be taken when practicing Pigeon Pose.

For lower back injuries, such as sciatica or herniated vertebral disks, Pigeon Pose should be modified.

⊕ Modifications and props

If the lower back is injured, move into this asana slowly and support the body by placing a yoga block or folded blanket underneath the right hip.

For knee injuries, place the right foot closer to the hips, so the bent knee is less extended, and place a yoga block or folded blanket underneath the right hip for support.

⊘ Try to

Lengthen the left leg, so the stretch is felt in the hip flexors of the back leg.

Keep the body's weight centered to avoid stress on the joints.

Keep the right knee in-line with the right side of the pelvis. This will make sure there is an effective stretch through the gluteal muscles.

⊗ Try not to

Avoid dropping the heel of the back foot out to the side, and instead stretch the toes back until a stretch is felt across the top of the ankle.

Avoid positioning the right foot forward to the point where discomfort is felt in the right knee.

How to do it

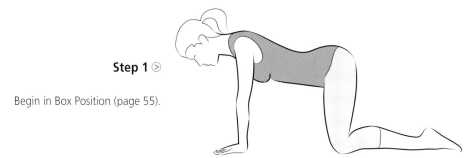

Step 1 ⊗

Begin in Box Position (page 55).

⊗ **Step 2**

Breathing deeply, transfer more of the body's weight into the arms and move the right knee to just behind the right wrist. Now slowly move the right foot over to the left side, so the right lower leg is laying diagonally across the floor. Flex the right ankle so the toes are moving toward the shin; this will help to protect the right knee.

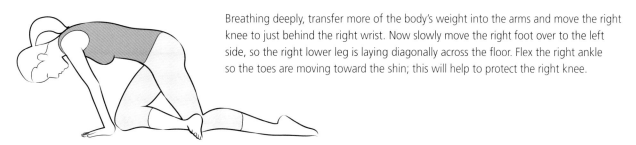

Step 3 ⊗

Exhale while extending the left leg back, so the left knee joint straightens and the hips move toward the ground. On an inhale, move the hands to each side of the right leg and extend the spine upward. The shoulders should be moving down, away from the ears, and the chin should be level with the ground.

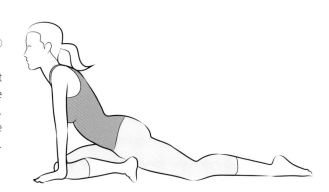

⊗ **Step 4**

Exhale and move the upper body forward at the same time, so it is positioned over the front leg, and rest the forearms on the ground in front of the right leg. Keep breathing deeply while the left leg extends back, so the hips sink farther toward the ground. Keep the shoulders relaxed and bring the gaze toward the ground in front of the hands.

Pigeon Pose

Eka Pada Kapotasana

During Pigeon Pose, the right femur externally rotates to the side, and the right knee is in a flexed position, with the lower leg on the ground. This position creates an eccentric lengthening of the quadriceps and gluteus minimus, medius, and maximus, and a concentric contraction of the hamstring. The tibialis anterior concentrically shortens, creating a dorsiflexion at the right ankle, while the soleus lengthens. The left leg is completely extended and the quadriceps shorten concentrically. The hip flexors, in particular, the rectus femoris, lengthen and extend to allow for the movement in the hip. The gluteus maximus also concentrically contracts on the left side, helping to extend the hip joint. The spine is in forward flexion with the quadratus lumborum lengthening eccentrically and the pelvis tilting forward. Pigeon pose also involves the iliopsoas concentrically shortening on the right side as the upper body moves toward the thigh, and eccentrically lengthening on the left side.

Anatomy of the pose

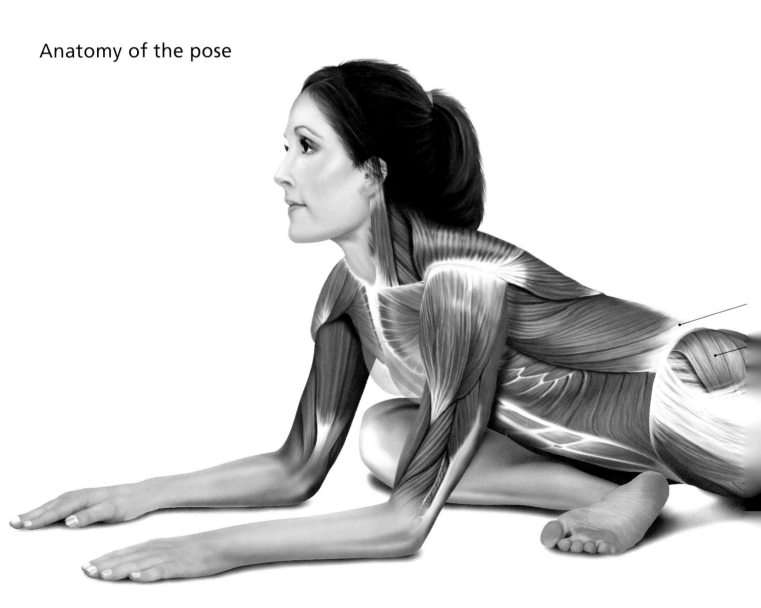

muscle activity

prime mover

1 Quadriceps (left leg)
2 Tibialis anterior (right leg)
3 Hamstrings

antagonist

4 Gluteus maximus,
  minimus, and medius
5 Rectus femoris
6 Iliopsoas
7 Quadratus lumborum

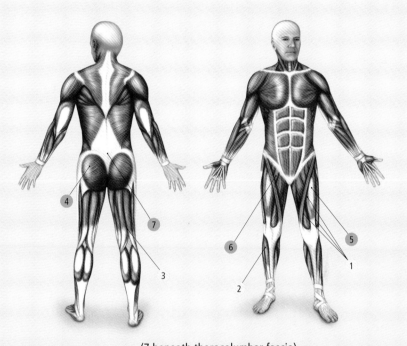

(7 beneath thoracolumbar fascia)

spine

The spine is in a forward flexed position in a sagittal plane, moving from a frontal axis.
The pelvis is in an anterior tilt position.

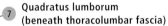

7 Quadratus lumborum
(beneath thoracolumbar fascia)

4 Gluteus maximus, minimus,
and medius

Not visible from this view:
6 Iliopsoas (inside hip area, deep)
2 Tibialis anterior (lower leg)

3 Hamstrings

1 Quadriceps

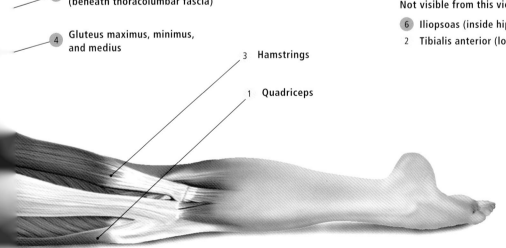

Wheel Pose

Urdhva Dhanurasana

Wheel Pose is an advanced asana that is the culmination of proficiency in more basic yoga asanas. Some flexibility of the shoulders, hips, and spine is required to perform it, but the mobility of all these joints is greatly improved with regular practice. The majority of the movement comes from the thoracic region of the spine, which moves into a deep bend, with the back muscles contracting powerfully and shortening. This greatly stretches the abdominal muscles and opens the whole of the upper body, including the front of the rib cage. The arms are completely extended, helping to stretch the shoulder joints and open the chest area. This then allows for the spine to move into a deep extension. The feet are positioned hips' width apart and the legs also extend, stretching the front of the hips, lengthening the hip flexors, and strengthening the quadriceps. The gluteal muscles contract to support the pelvis and lower back. The overall effect is increased flexibility and stability of the shoulders, hips, and spine.

Level

Advanced

Benefits

Wheel Pose stretches the entire upper body and increases the range of movement of the spine, shoulders, and hips.

It strengthens the arms and legs, energizes the whole body, and is mentally uplifting.

Caution

People with back or shoulder injuries or high blood pressure should be careful when practicing Wheel Pose.

⊕ Modifications and props

For high blood pressure and more severe back injuries, Shoulder Bridge Pose is a more appropriate asana.

For shoulder injuries, face away from a wall with about 20 in. (50 cm) space between the wall and the heels. Stretch the arms up overhead and reach the hands back until they can be placed flat onto the wall and the spine arches a little. Practice this modification until the injury heals, before moving into full Wheel Pose.

Try to

Open the chest area by pressing firmly into the hands, extending the elbow joints and letting the neck relax.

Work the gluteal muscles without tightening them too much, because this can put undue pressure on the bottom of the spine.

Keep the elbows in-line with the shoulders to be sure of maximum support from the triceps.

Try not to

Avoid compressing the lower back; keep the legs firm and lengthen the spine. Focus on opening the chest by pressing firmly into the hands and gently pushing the chest forward. This action will help create a more even bend along the spine, as opposed to just bending from the lower back.

How to do it

Step 1 ⊙

Begin by lying face up with the legs bent and the feet flat on the ground. The arms should be resting by the sides of the body. The breath is slow and steady.

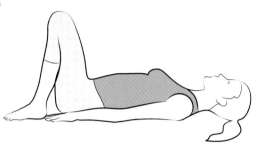

⊙ Step 2

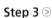

Inhale while placing the hands on the ground on each side of the neck, with the fingers pointing toward the shoulders. The elbows should be bent with the whole hands, including the palms and heels, on the ground. Stretch out the fingers and thumbs and relax the toes.

Step 3 ⊙

Now exhale deeply while pressing firmly into the hands and feet, so the legs and arms begin to extend and straighten, lifting the spine and hips from the ground. The front of the rib cage should move up, creating an arch in the spine. The knees and elbows should still be partly bent, with the head hovering just above the ground.

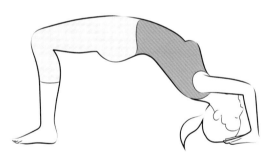

⊙ Step 4

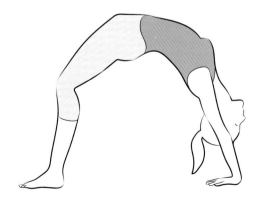

Breathe steadily and completely extend the arms and legs without compressing the lower back. Keep the elbows in-line with the shoulders and the knees in-line with the ankles. Press firmly into the feet and lift the hips upward. Relax the gluteal muscles a little and try to relax the upper body, letting the chest open and stretch. Relax the neck and head and keep the gaze parallel to the ground, as opposed to looking at the ground.

Wheel Pose

Urdhva Dhanurasana

Wheel pose is an intense backbending position that deeply stretches the chest and abdominal area and strengthens all the muscles surrounding the spine. The arms are straight and completely extended at the shoulder and elbow joint. The triceps contract concentrically and the deltoids lengthen eccentrically to let the shoulder joint open. The muscles of the back, including the erector spinae and latissimus dorsi, concentrically contract powerfully to move the spine into an extended position. The opposing muscle groups, including the pectoral muscles, rectus abdominis, and transversus abdominis, all lengthen eccentrically, allowing for the upper body to open and stretch. The hip flexors eccentrically lengthen and the gluteus maximus muscles are in a concentric contraction, extending the hip joint. The knees are in partial flexion because of a concentric contraction of the quadriceps, which are working to stabilize the knee joint.

muscle activity

prime mover

1   Erector spinae
2   Latissimus dorsi
3   Gluteus maximus
4   Quadriceps
5   Deltoids

antagonist

6   Rectus abdominis
7   Transversus abdominis
8   Hip flexors
9   Pectoralis major and minor

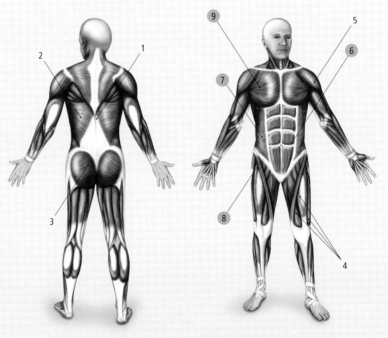

(1 beneath thoracolumbar fascia)

spine

The spine is in an extended position and moves on a sagittal plane from a frontal axis.
The pelvis is in a posterior tilt position.

Anatomy of the pose

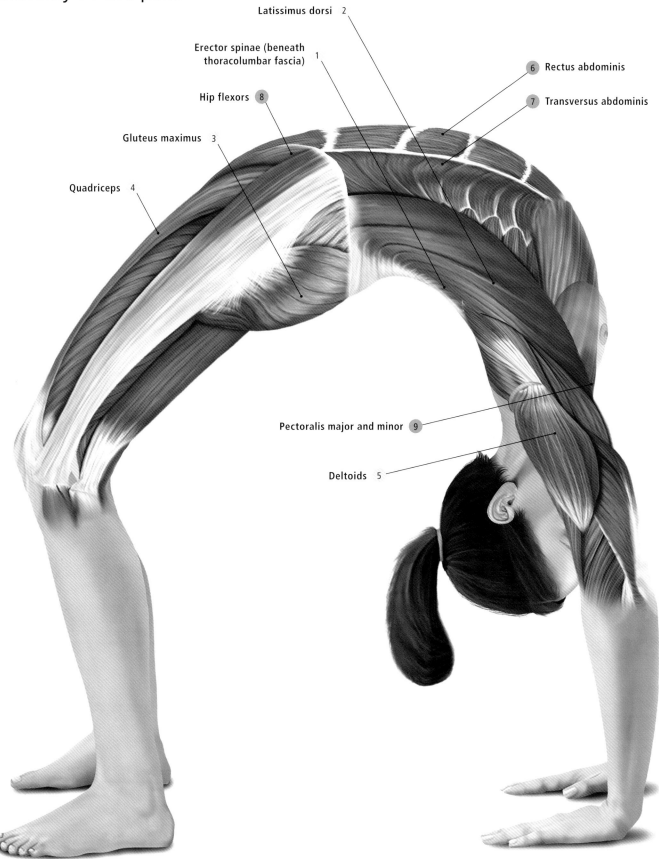

Latissimus dorsi 2

Erector spinae (beneath thoracolumbar fascia) 1

Hip flexors 8

Gluteus maximus 3

Quadriceps 4

6 Rectus abdominis

7 Transversus abdominis

Pectoralis major and minor 9

Deltoids 5

Cat Pose to Cow Pose

Marjariasana to Bitilasana

Cat Pose and Cow Pose are gentle asanas that are often performed together (as shown here) and that improve the flexibility of the spine, in particular, the thoracic region. During Cat Pose, the muscles of the back are stretched while the abdominal muscles are contracted. This action gently massages the abdominal organs. During Cow Pose, the muscles of the back contract while the abdominal muscles stretch. By increasing the mobility of the spine in this way, not only are the front and back muscles of the torso both stretched and strengthened, but it is thought that synovial fluid is released to circulate around the vertebrae and blood flow through the muscles, and, therefore, the spinal disks, is increased.

For both Cat and Cow Pose, place the hands with the palms flat to the ground, stretching the wrist flexors. This weight-bearing action gradually increases bone density and, therefore, strengthens the wrists. This then makes the wrist flexibility required for asanas like Wheel Pose more attainable.

Level

Beginner

Benefits

Cat and Cow Pose increase the flexibility of the spine, surrounding muscles, and connective tissue, resulting in a decreased likelihood of back pain.

Flexibility and strength of the wrists is also increased.

Caution

Those with wrist or knee injuries may need to modify this asana.

For neck injuries, including whiplash, maintain neutral alignment of the neck when practicing Cow Pose.

⊕ Modifications and props

If the knees are injured, place a folded blanket under them for cushioning. If it is not possible to bend the wrists in this way, the arms can be extended, in-line with the back, and placed on a chair in front of the head.

⊘ Try to

When moving into Cat Pose, try to create space across the middle of the back by arching from the middle of the spine and drawing the crown of the head and coccyx downward.

For Cow Pose, elongate from the lower back to the neck and aim for a stretch across the front of the rib cage, while keeping the shoulders down away from the ears.

⊗ Try not to

For Cat Pose, avoid applying a lot of weight to the wrists and instead gently contract the muscles of the torso so that the whole body is working.

When in Cow Pose, avoid overextending the neck and lower back to the point where pressure is felt in these areas. Instead, aim for a sense of length through the neck and lumbar spine, and bend as far as is comfortable.

How to do it

Step 1 ⊘

Begin in Box Position (page 55).

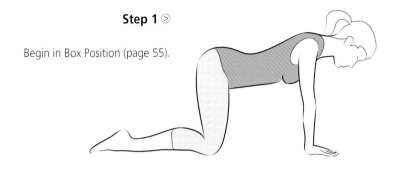

⊘ **Step 2**

To move into Cat Pose, exhale deeply while rounding the spine, moving initially from the center of the back. The coccyx should point toward the ground, as should the crown of the head, and the chin should move in toward the chest. The scapulae move away from one another and the abdominal muscles contract and move in toward the spine. The entire back area is being lengthened and stretched and is now in a concave position.

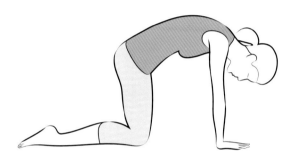

Step 3 ⊘

Pause before moving into Cow Pose. Inhale to sink the thoracic spine down as the tailbone and crown of the head move upward. The shoulders should be drawn down away from the ears and the front of the torso lengthened from the chin to the navel. The muscles of the back should contract as the front torso muscles lengthen and stretch. The spine is now in a convex position.

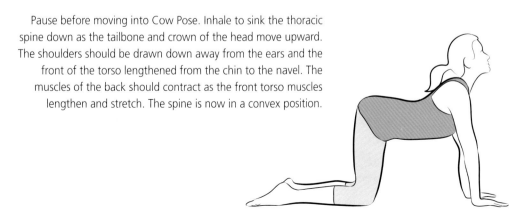

Cat Pose to Cow Pose

Marjariasana to Bitilasana

In the start position for Cat Pose, the triceps concentrically contract to make the arms extend, and the iliopsoas muscles shorten and partly flex the hip so the thighs are perpendicular to the ground. During Cat Pose, the spine moves into a convex position, which is achieved when the rectus abdominis and transversus abdominis concentrically contract. This leads to a rounding of the thoracic region of the spine, in which the oblique abdominal muscles assist. The pectoral and anterior deltoid muscles also shorten via a concentric contraction to help round the upper back. To allow for this articulation of the spine, the erector spinae muscles lengthen eccentrically, and the trapezius muscles stretch to move the scapulae into "prostration," moving them away from one another. Other muscles of the back that lengthen eccentrically include the splenius capitis, splenius cervicis, and latissimus dorsi.

When moving into Cow Pose, the main muscle groups that lengthen and shorten are effectively reversed to let the spine move into a concave position.

NB: The prime movers in Cat Pose become the antagonists when moving into Cow Pose, and vice versa:

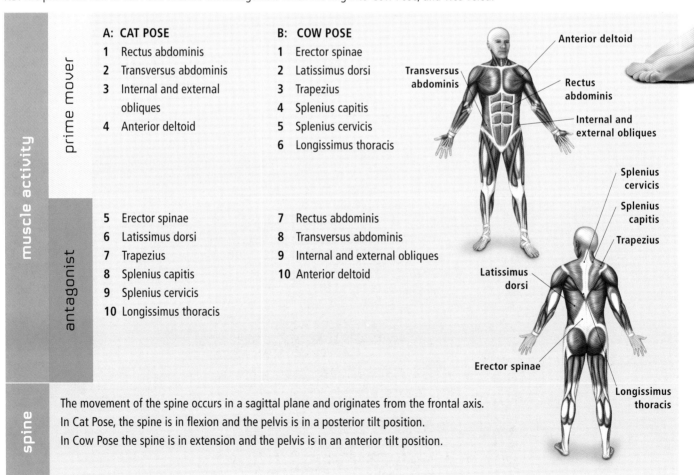

muscle activity

prime mover

A: CAT POSE
1 Rectus abdominis
2 Transversus abdominis
3 Internal and external obliques
4 Anterior deltoid

B: COW POSE
1 Erector spinae
2 Latissimus dorsi
3 Trapezius
4 Splenius capitis
5 Splenius cervicis
6 Longissimus thoracis

antagonist

5 Erector spinae
6 Latissimus dorsi
7 Trapezius
8 Splenius capitis
9 Splenius cervicis
10 Longissimus thoracis

7 Rectus abdominis
8 Transversus abdominis
9 Internal and external obliques
10 Anterior deltoid

spine

The movement of the spine occurs in a sagittal plane and originates from the frontal axis.
In Cat Pose, the spine is in flexion and the pelvis is in a posterior tilt position.
In Cow Pose the spine is in extension and the pelvis is in an anterior tilt position.

Anatomy of the pose

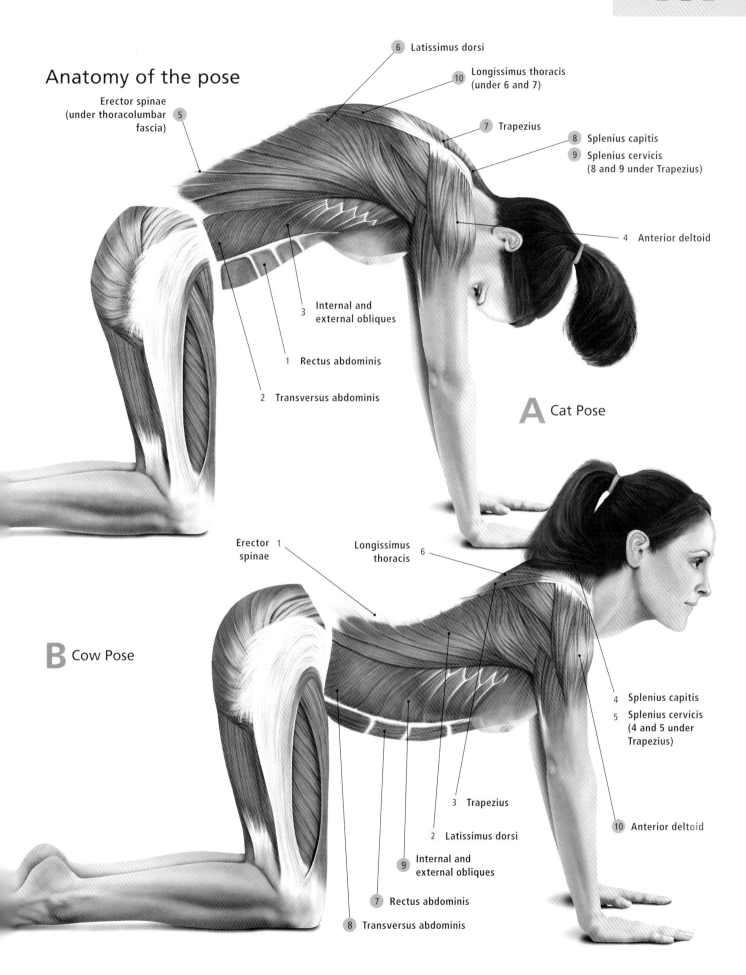

6 Latissimus dorsi

10 Longissimus thoracis (under 6 and 7)

Erector spinae (under thoracolumbar fascia) 5

7 Trapezius

8 Splenius capitis

9 Splenius cervicis (8 and 9 under Trapezius)

4 Anterior deltoid

3 Internal and external obliques

1 Rectus abdominis

2 Transversus abdominis

A Cat Pose

B Cow Pose

Erector spinae 1

Longissimus thoracis 6

4 Splenius capitis

5 Splenius cervicis (4 and 5 under Trapezius)

10 Anterior deltoid

3 Trapezius

2 Latissimus dorsi

9 Internal and external obliques

7 Rectus abdominis

8 Transversus abdominis

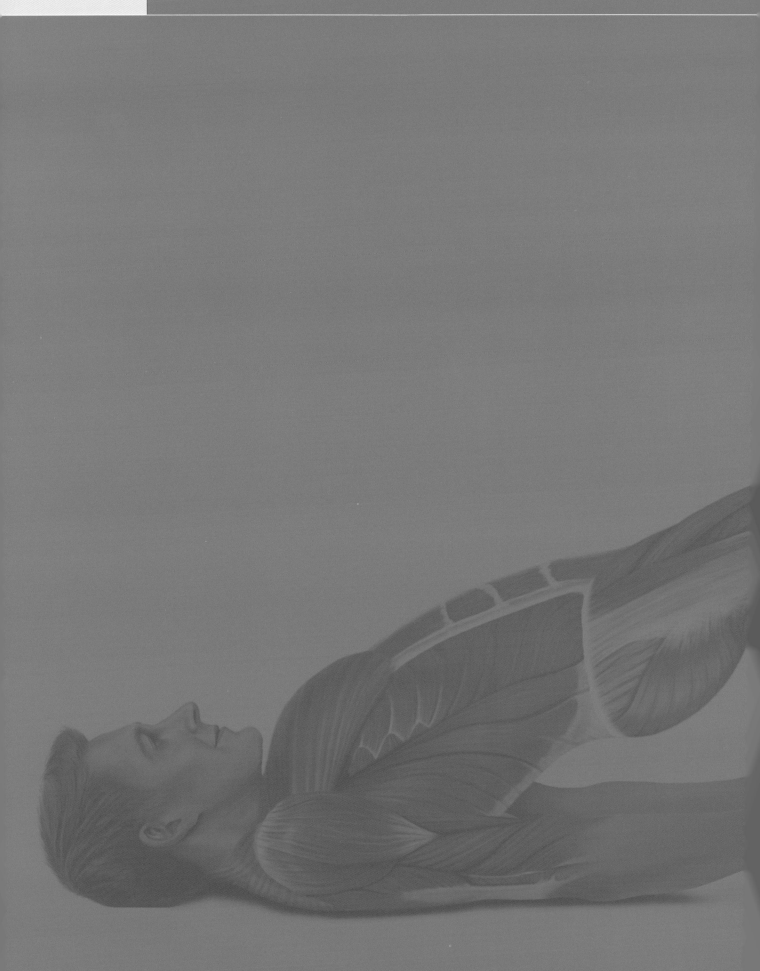

Inversions

Inversions involve the head being positioned lower than the heart. There are two distinct groups of inversions: one is relatively calming and includes Shoulder Stand Pose and Downward-Facing Dog Pose; the other is more stimulating and includes Headstand Pose. The latter type can help people overcome emotional blocks, such as fear and lack of confidence. The overall effect of any inversion is improved circulation and renewed oxygen to the brain, thus increasing mental concentration and memory.

Downward-Facing Dog Pose

Adho Mukha Svanasana

Downward-Facing Dog Pose is a fundamental pose that is sometimes used as a resting asana in between more challenging poses. The arms are straight with the hands pressed into the ground and the fingers and thumbs spread out with the middle finger pointing directly forward. This helps minimize pressure in the wrist joint. This action also strengthens the arms and stretches the shoulder joints and chest, while the muscles of the upper back contract to keep the shoulder blades in the correct alignment.

The spine is in a neutral position and there is an emphasis on lengthening the entire spine, from the sacrum to the neck, and on creating space around the rib cage as well. The legs are straight, with the thighs firm, and the calf muscles lengthen as the heels move toward the ground, increasing flexibility in the ankle joints. The pelvis is tilted forward, so the seat bones and coccyx move upward, stretching the backs of the legs even farther. This also enables the lower back and gluteal muscles to stretch more, helping to relieve lower back pain.

Level

Beginner

Benefits

This asana opens the shoulders and lengthens the muscles along the spine.

It stretches the hamstrings and calf muscles and opens the shoulders, improving overall postural alignment.

Caution

People with low blood pressure may find this is affected when Downward-Facing Dog Pose is held for extended periods of time.

Those with wrist injuries should be cautious when practicing this asana.

⊕ Modifications and props

To modify this asana, remain on the knees with the hips aligned over the knees. Extend the arms forward and sink the chest to the floor, resting the forehead on the ground.

For neck injuries, Downward-Facing Dog Pose can be practiced with a yoga block underneath the top of the head to support the neck.

⊘ Try to

Lengthen through the spine by pressing firmly into the hands and moving the hips upward before dropping the heels to the floor and moving the hips back a little.

Relax the neck and move the shoulders away from the head to create space around the neck.

⊗ Try not to

Avoid forcing the heels to the floor, because this may strain the Achilles tendon. Instead, aim for a gentle stretch in the shoulder joint by pressing into the hands, and let the heels slowly drop toward the ground.

How to do it

Step 1 ⊚

Begin in Box Position (page 55).

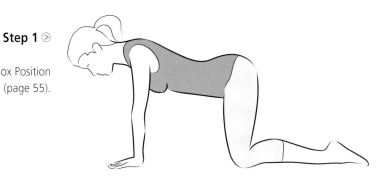

⊚ **Step 2**

Move the hands forward by about the length of one hand. Stretch the fingers out, making sure the middle finger is pointing forward. Tuck the toes under.

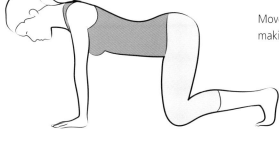

⊚ **Step 3**

Now inhale while pressing firmly into the hands and lifting the knees from the floor, gradually raising the hips upward. At first, keep the knees slightly bent and the heels lifted away from the ground. Focus on elongating the spine and lifting the seat bones upward. Keep pressing firmly into the hands and exhale deeply.

⊚ **Step 4**

Now let the heels drop toward the ground so the knee joints straighten. The arms, spine, and legs should now be straight. Gently contract the abdominal muscles and move the shoulder blades away from the head, keeping the neck relaxed. The gaze should be toward the lower legs. Breathe steadily.

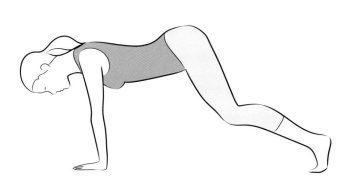

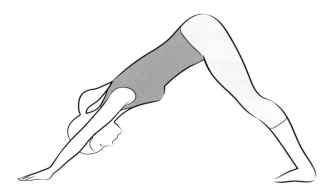

Downward-Facing Dog Pose

Adho Mukha Svanasana

In Downward-Facing Dog Pose, the arms and legs are extended, helping to stretch several major muscles groups, while the quadriceps shorten concentrically to extend the knees. The deltoid muscles lengthen eccentrically to extend the arms from the shoulder joint, and then internally rotate the upper arms, resulting in pronation of the forearms. This internal rotation leads to the stabilization of the shoulder girdle. There is a concentric contraction of the triceps, allowing for the biceps brachii to lengthen eccentrically and the elbow joint to completely extend. The trapezius muscles then contract concentrically to move the scapulae away from the head. The erector spinae is in an eccentric stretch while the iliopsoas shortens concentrically, so the hip joint is only partly flexed. With the pelvis at this angle, the gluteus maximus, hamstrings, soleus, and gastrocnemius all lengthen eccentrically. The ankle joint is in a dorsiflexed position brought about partly by a concentric contraction of tibialis anterior.

muscle activity

prime mover

1 Iliopsoas
2 Quadriceps
3 Trapezius
4 Tibialis anterior
5 Anterior deltoid

antagonist

6 Hamstrings
7 Erector spinae
8 Gluteus maximus
9 Soleus and gastrocnemius
10 Posterior deltoid

(7 beneath thoracolumbar fascia)

spine

The spine is in a neutral position, moving in a sagittal plane from a frontal axis.
The pelvis is in an anterior tilt position.

Anatomy of the pose

Not visible from this view:

1   Iliopsoas (inside hip area, deep)

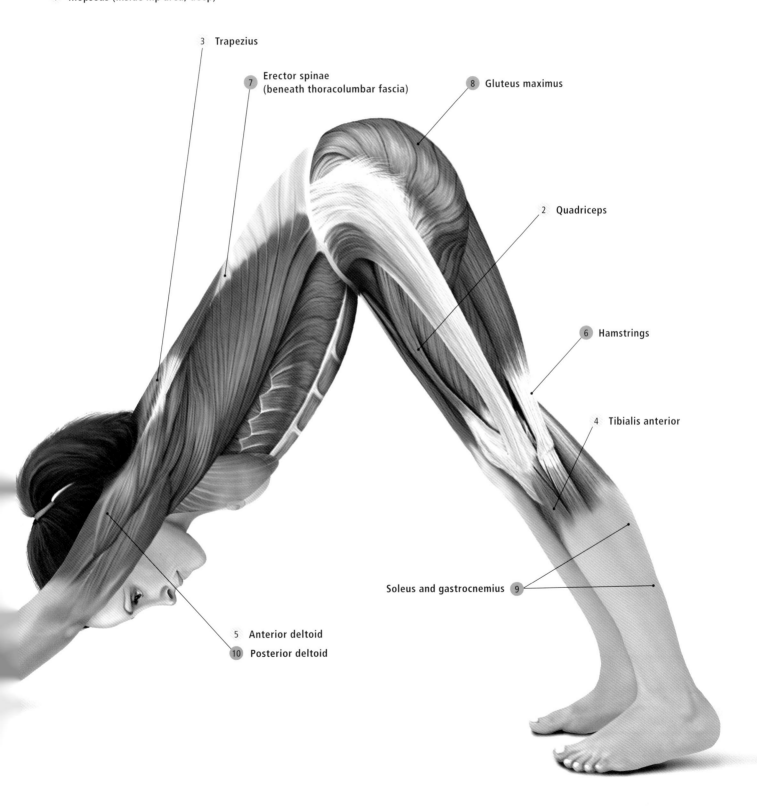

3   Trapezius

7   Erector spinae
(beneath thoracolumbar fascia)

8   Gluteus maximus

2   Quadriceps

6   Hamstrings

4   Tibialis anterior

Soleus and gastrocnemius   9

5   Anterior deltoid

10   Posterior deltoid

Shoulder Bridge Pose
Setu Bandhasana Sarvangasana

Shoulder Bridge Pose is one of the more gentle backbends. It strengthens the legs and back, and increases flexibility in the spine and shoulders. It is a useful asana to practice before more challenging postures, such as Wheel Pose, because it stretches the chest and shoulders and mobilizes the spine.

The knees are bent with the ankles aligned directly underneath the knees joints and the feet are hips' width apart. This position helps to avoid strain on the knee tendons and unnecessary tension in the gluteal muscles. The hips and spine are lifted from the ground until an arch is created through the entire spine. The arms are on the ground under the spine with the hands interlaced, moving the shoulder blades toward one another and the chest toward the chin. This helps to stretch the chest and the front of the shoulders and strengthens the extensor muscles of the spine. The legs are working hard to keep the knees in alignment with the hips, with the hamstrings and gluteal muscles contracting and the quadriceps lengthening so the knees can bend.

Level

Intermediate

Benefits

This asana strengthens the muscles of the spine, legs, and hips.

It increases the flexibility of the chest, shoulders, and spine and invigorates the whole body, increasing energy levels.

Caution

People with high blood pressure or neck or lower back injuries should be cautious with this asana.

⊕ Modifications and props

To modify the asana for either high blood pressure of back injuries, support the spine by placing a yoga brick or bolster underneath the lower back.

To avoid aggravating neck injuries, do not interlace the fingers under the back and instead rest the hands flat on the floor with the arms straight.

Try to

Keep the knees in-line with the front hip bones and try to draw the shoulder blades toward one another to create more lift through the chest and spine.

Try not to

Try not to lift the hips to a position where there is pressure on the spine.

Do not allow the knees to be wider apart than the ankles, because this will put strain on the knee joints.

Avoid pressing into the heels and lifting the toes; instead, relax the toes, because this will help to minimize tension in the lower back.

How to do it

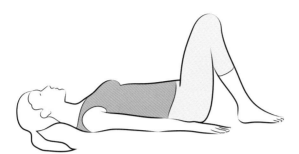

⊘ Step 1

Begin by lying face up with the legs bent, feet flat on the floor and hips' width apart.

Step 2 ⊙

The knees should be aligned directly over the ankles. The arms should be resting on the ground on each side of the body, with the palms of the hands facing down. Keeping the head and neck still and the feet flat on the ground, exhale as the hips and spine lift away from the ground. There should now be a diagonal straight line from the knees to the shoulders with the spine in a neutral position.

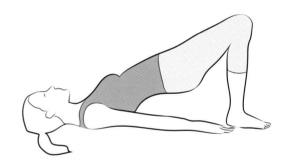

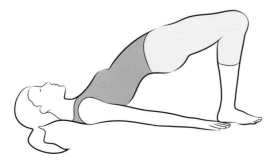

⊘ Step 3

Now inhale while lifting the pelvis higher, so the chest moves toward the chin and the spine is in a slight backbending position, creating an arch through the middle back. Keep breathing steadily and move the shoulder blades back toward one another while simultaneously moving the arms toward one another, underneath the back. Interlace the fingers underneath the back. Contract the muscles of the lower body, including the gluteal muscles, hamstrings, and lower abdominal muscles.

Shoulder Bridge Pose

Setu Bandhasana Sarvangasana

During Shoulder Bridge Pose, the hamstrings concentrically contract, flexing the knees. This creates an eccentric lengthening of the quadriceps and hip flexor muscle groups, which then work as fixators, holding the femurs in place. The gluteus maximus muscles also contract concentrically and support both the pelvis and sacroiliac joint. The spine, mainly the thoracic region, is in an extended position that is created when the quadratus lumborum and erector spinae muscles contract concentrically. By moving the hips upward to the full Shoulder Bridge position, the pectoral and anterior deltoid muscles eccentrically lengthen, and the trapezius muscles contract concentrically to retract the scapulae toward the spine, moving the sternum closer to the chin. The ankle joints are in neutral, with the feet flat to the ground.

Anatomy of the pose

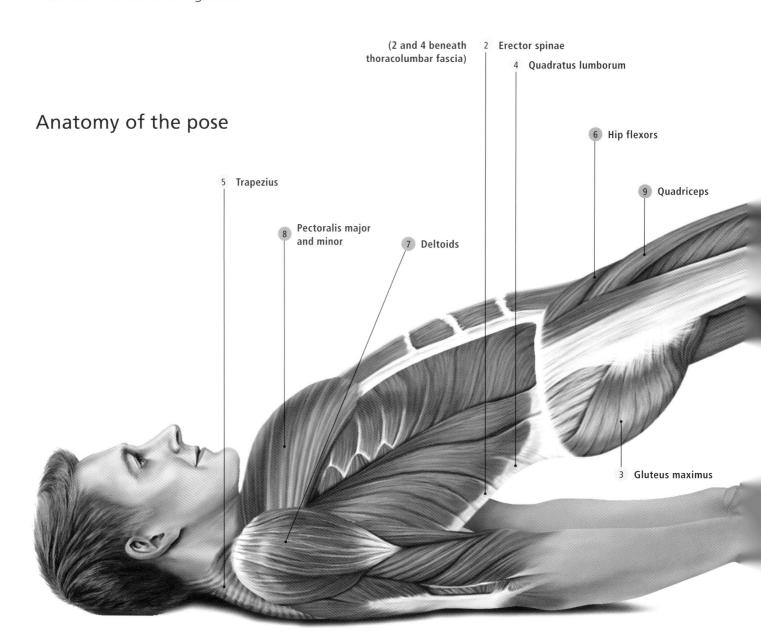

(2 and 4 beneath thoracolumbar fascia)

2   Erector spinae

4   Quadratus lumborum

6   Hip flexors

5   Trapezius

9   Quadriceps

8   Pectoralis major and minor

7   Deltoids

3   Gluteus maximus

muscle activity

prime mover

1 Hamstrings
2 Erector spinae
3 Gluteus maximus
4 Quadratus lumborum
5 Trapezius

antagonist

6 Hip flexors
7 Deltoids
8 Pectoralis major and minor
9 Quadriceps

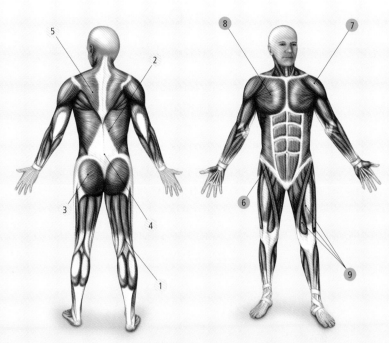

(2 and 4 beneath thoracolumbar fascia)

spine

The spine is in an extended position and moves in a sagittal plane from a frontal axis.
The pelvis is in an anterior tilt position.

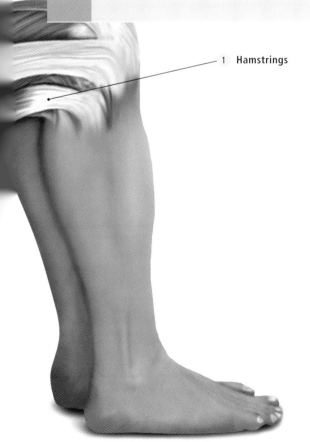

1 Hamstrings

Shoulder Stand Pose

Sarvangasana

It can take some time before a person practicing yoga is ready for Shoulder Stand Pose, because it requires strength and flexibility of all the major joints. It is an inversion asana, meaning that the head is lower than the heart, and strengthens the whole body and improves respiratory function.

The weight of the body is placed mainly on the shoulders, with the chin tucked in toward the chest, which stretches the neck. The elbows should be bent with the hands resting lightly on the middle of the back to support the upper body. The spine should lengthen upward in a straight line, which requires the spinal extensors to stretch and the abdominal muscles to contract to help maintain the position. The legs and feet should also stretch upward and press firmly together. The chest and front of the shoulders stretch while the upper back and back of the shoulders contract to move the shoulder blades together. This allows for the person to move onto the tops of the shoulders and straighten the spine more effectively.

Level

Intermediate

Benefits

Shoulder Stand Pose strengthens the muscles of the back and abdomen and increases the flexibility of the shoulders and spine.

The thyroid gland and abdominal organs are stimulated, improving metabolism. This asana strengths the heart and lungs, which, in turn, improves respiratory function.

Caution

People with neck injuries or high blood pressure should not practice Shoulder Stand Pose.

Those with shoulder or back injuries should practice with caution.

⊕ Modifications and props

To modify Shoulder Stand Pose, lie on the back with the knees bent and the soles of the feet on a wall, so the lower legs are parallel to the ground. Push the feet firmly against the wall and lift the hips and spine away from the ground until the knees, hips, and shoulders create one straight line. Place the hands on the back for support, keeping the feet on the wall for additional support.

⊙ Try to

Reach the feet upward to create more length through the body and press the legs together firmly, creating a sense of strength though the lower body.

Stretch across the chest area by moving the elbows toward one another. This will also move the body's weight away from the neck and onto the shoulders.

⊗ Try not to

The chin must stay in-line with the sternum, so avoid moving the head, because this can injure the neck.

Do not let the weight of the hips rest on the hands; instead work toward straightening the spine and creating a feeling of lift through the body.

How to do it

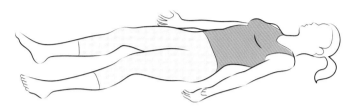

⊘ **Step 1**

Begin in Corpse Pose (page 55).

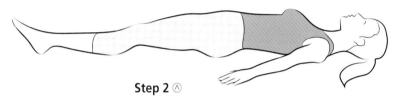

Step 2 ⌃

Move the arms toward the sides of the upper body, with the palms of the hands facing down, and press the legs together.

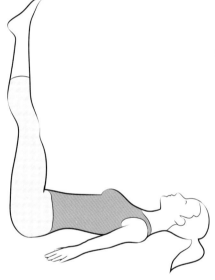

⌃ **Step 3**

Contract the abdominal muscles on an exhale and lift the legs until they are perpendicular to the ground. The hips should still be on the ground and the body should now be at a right angle.

⊘ **Step 4**

On an inhale, reach the legs upward and straighten the spine, so the hips are aligned directly over the shoulders. On an exhale, move the hands closer to the shoulder blades and move the elbows a little closer together. This will help open the front of the shoulders and chest, moving the hips into a more neutral alignment. Reach the feet upward, stretching all the way to the toes. Make sure the breath is calm and steady.

Shoulder Stand Pose

Sarvangasana

During Shoulder Stand Pose, the cervical spine is in forward flexion, while the lumbar and thoracic spine is in a neutral position. The shoulders, pelvis, knees, and ankles are all in alignment. To move the spine into this position, the latissimus dorsi and erector spinae muscles initially stretch eccentrically, then contract concentrically, and finally isometrically to stabilize the upper body. The rectus abdominis also helps to stabilize the upper body, acting as a fixator muscle. The pelvis is in a neutral alignment and the legs are completely extended away from the hips. This position occurs when the gluteus maximus contracts concentrically and the hip flexors lengthen eccentrically. The knees are then completely extended and the quadriceps and hamstrings are in an isometric contraction, fixating the legs in this extended position. The ankle joints plantar flex the feet when the gastrocnemius and soleus shorten via a concentric contraction. To move the arms into the flexed position, the anterior deltoids, pectoral muscles, and triceps all lengthen eccentrically and the biceps brachii, trapezius, and posterior deltoids all shorten concentrically.

muscle activity

prime mover

1 Latissimus dorsi
2 Quadriceps
3 Gastrocnemius
4 Biceps brachii
5 Gluteus maximus
6 Deltoids

antagonist

7 Hamstrings
8 Erector spinae
9 Pectoralis major and minor

(8 beneath thoracolumbar fascia)

spine

The thoracic and lumbar areas of the spine are in a neutral position, and the cervical spine is in forward flexion.
The spine moves in a sagittal plane from a frontal axis.
The pelvis is also in a neutral position.

Anatomy of the pose

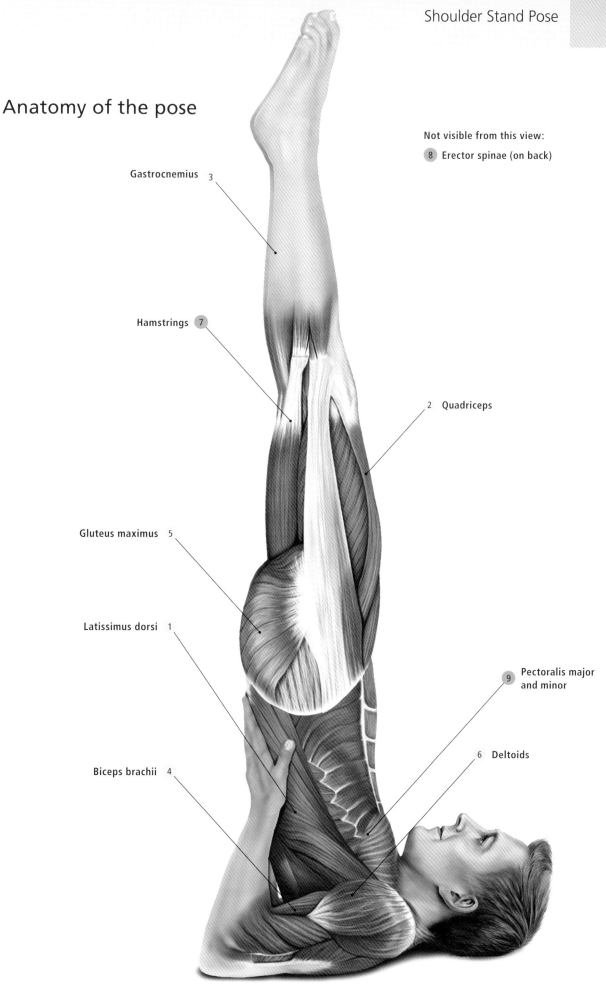

Gastrocnemius 3

Hamstrings 7

Gluteus maximus 5

Latissimus dorsi 1

Biceps brachii 4

Not visible from this view:
8 Erector spinae (on back)

2 Quadriceps

9 Pectoralis major and minor

6 Deltoids

Plow Pose

Halasana

Plow Pose is an inverted asana, meaning the head is lower than the heart, which increases circulation and invigorates the whole body. It should be practiced toward the end of a yoga session, when the body is completely warmed up and already stretched, to avoid injury. It stimulates the thyroid, adrenal, and pituitary glands by compressing the front of the upper body, which helps to balance the metabolic system.

Several major muscle groups are stretched, leading to improved flexibility of the spine, shoulders, and legs. The spinal extensor muscles are lengthened and the muscles of the neck deeply stretched. The arms are completely straightened, which stretches the biceps brachii and the front of the shoulders. The muscles of the upper back, mainly the trapezius, contract to draw the shoulder blades together. This, in turn, stretches the chest area, helping to improve posture. The legs are straight and the toes are tucked under, which stretches the hamstring and calf muscles.

Level

Intermediate

Benefits

The whole spine is stretched in Plow Pose, increasing the flexibility of the upper body.

The compression through the front of the upper body stimulates the thyroid gland and abdominal organs, which, in turn, stimulates the digestive system.

Caution

People with neck injuries and high blood pressure should avoid Plow Pose.

Those with lower back injuries should also practice with caution.

⊕ Modifications and props

If the full asana is too intense, keep the hands on the middle of the back and rest the feet on a bolster or some yoga blocks, so the stretch of the spine is lessened.

⊘ Try to

Create space in the upper body by lengthening the spine.

Move the shoulder blades toward one another by stretching the arms away from the body, increasing the stretch across the chest and front of the shoulders.

Always keep the head and neck still in Plow Pose to avoid injury.

⊗ Try not to

Avoid rounding the spine and instead straighten the back by moving the hips upward, creating a straight line from the shoulders to the hips.

Let the chin move toward the chest, but avoid placing undue strain on the neck. If the neck is uncomfortable, slowly move out of the asana and rest.

How to do it

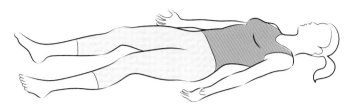

⊲ **Step 1**

Begin in Corpse Pose (page 55).

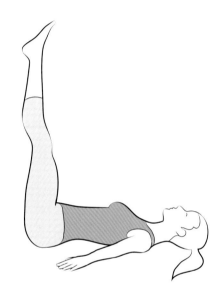

Step 2 ⊳

Move the arms toward the sides of the upper body, with the palms of the hands facing down, and press the legs together. On an exhale, contract the abdominal muscles and lift the legs until they are perpendicular to the ground. The hips should still be on the ground and the body should now be at a right angle.

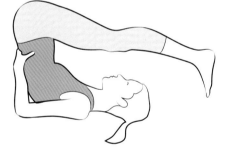

⊼ **Step 3**

Press firmly into the hands and inhale while lifting the hips and spine from the floor. Breathe evenly and move slowly until the spine is straightened, with the hips aligned over the shoulders. The legs should now be parallel to the floor. Bend the elbows and place the hands on the middle of the back to support the upper body.

⊽ **Step 4**

With the legs straight, bring the feet to the ground and tuck the toes under so the heels are aligned over the balls of the feet. Contract the thigh muscles and now bring the arms straight onto the ground. On an exhale, stretch the front of the shoulders by interlacing the hands and completely extending the arms.

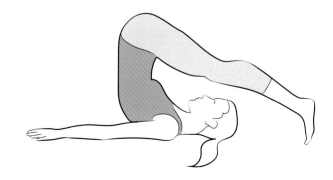

Plow Pose

Halasana

In Plow Pose, the major muscle groups of the back, erector spinae and latissimus dorsi, lengthen eccentrically while the hip flexors, mainly the iliopsoas, contract concentrically to move the legs toward the torso. The gluteus maximus also stretches eccentrically to increase the angle at the back of the pelvis. This action moves the spine into a neutral position and the hips into a partly flexed position. The triceps contract concentrically and the arms are completely extended with the forearms pronated. This results in an eccentric stretch of the pectoral muscles and anterior deltoids, and a concentric contraction of the posterior deltoids and trapezius muscles. The hamstrings lengthen eccentrically and the quadriceps contract concentrically, which completely extends the knee joints. The ankles are in dorsiflexion, stretching the soleus and gastrocnemius muscles. The neck is in forward flexion.

Anatomy of the pose

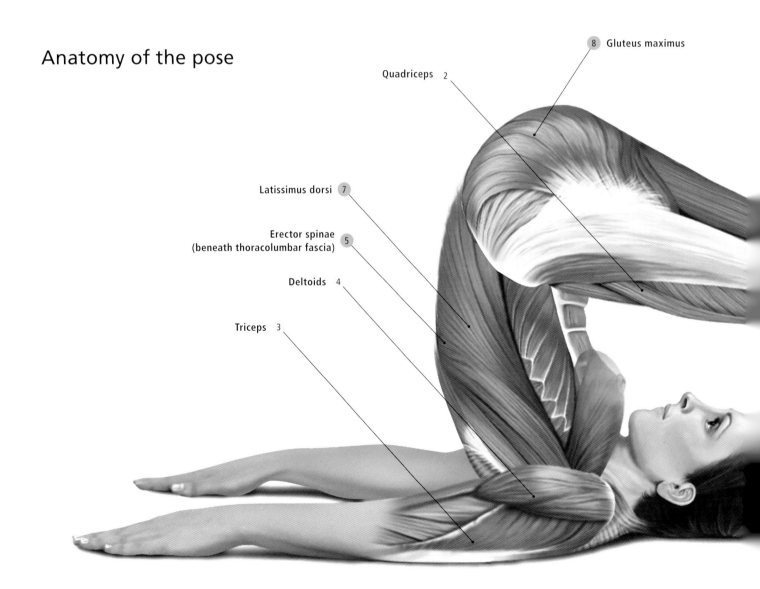

8 Gluteus maximus

Quadriceps   2

Latissimus dorsi   7

Erector spinae
(beneath thoracolumbar fascia)   5

Deltoids   4

Triceps   3

muscle activity

prime mover

1 Iliopsoas
2 Quadriceps
3 Triceps
4 Deltoids

antagonist

5 Erector spinae
6 Hamstrings
7 Latissimus dorsi
8 Gluteus maximus

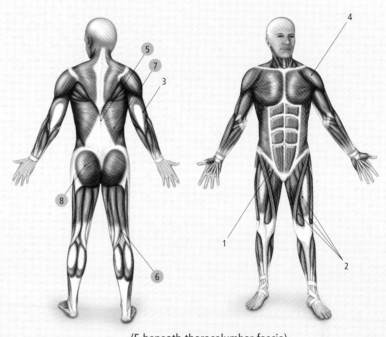

(5 beneath thoracolumbar fascia)

spine

The lumbar and thoracic spine regions should be in a neutral position and the cervical spine in forward flexion. The spine moves in a sagittal plane from a frontal axis. The pelvis is in a slight posterior tilt.

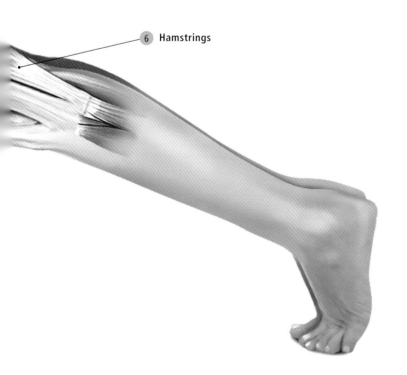

6 Hamstrings

Not visible from this view:

1 Iliopsoas (inside hip area, deep)

Headstand Pose

Shirshasana

Headstand Pose is one of the more challenging inversions within the yoga system and has many benefits. By inverting the body in this way, blood flows to the brain while gravity stimulates the blood's return in the veins, improving overall circulation. The respiratory rate is also increased, which helps to strengthen the lungs, improving overall well-being.

All the major muscles groups work hard to stabilize the body and maintain balance. The arms are bent with the fingers and thumbs firmly interlaced, while the muscles across the upper back move the shoulder blades away from the head and neck. This creates a strong framework for the head and neck area. The core muscles, namely the rectus and transversus abdominis, and the lower back muscles help to hold the spine in place. The legs are completely extended from the hips, with the gluteal and hip flexor muscles supporting the pelvis. The legs press together powerfully with the feet stretching upward, giving the sense of strength and lift through the whole body.

Level

Advanced

Benefits

This asana is invigorating and rejuvenating. It strengthens the shoulders and upper back muscles, in particular, as well as greatly improving core stability.

Regular practice of Headstand Pose also helps to build self-confidence.

Caution

For those with high blood pressure or neck or shoulder injuries, Headstand Pose should not be practiced.

⊕ Modifications and props

To modify this asana, remain at stage three and practice aligning the hips over the shoulders. When ready to move up into a complete headstand, first use a wall for support (facing away from the wall) while getting used to lifting the legs.

Try to

Create space for the neck by working powerfully across the upper back and by pressing the forearms into the ground.

From the legs, imagine the feet are being gently pulled upward, creating a sense of lift through the entire body.

Keep the spine in a neutral position by flattening the lower back area so the front of the rib cage draws in, as though moving in toward the middle spine.

Try not to

Avoid resting on the head; instead, contract the trapezius muscles, so the upper back and shoulder joints create support for the head and neck.

Avoid arching the lower back area, because this puts pressure on the vertebral disks.

Never move the head or neck while in this position, because injury may occur.

How to do it

⊗ Step 1

Begin in Box Position (page 55).

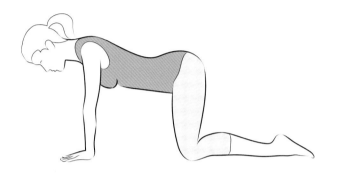

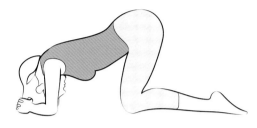

⊗ Step 2

Place the forearms on the ground, keeping the elbows at shoulders' width apart. Now interlace the fingers and thumbs tightly and press the little-finger edges of the hands firmly onto the ground. The palms of the hands should not be pressed together. Move the knees about 8 in. (20 cm) closer to the arms and place the back of the head into the palms of the hands and the crown of the head lightly onto the ground. The spine should be rounded at this point.

Step 3 ⊗

Tuck the toes under and, with the feet still on the ground, exhale and straighten the legs. Move the feet closer to the upper body until the hips are aligned directly over the shoulders. The spine should now be straight. Now move the shoulders away from the head by working the upper back and shoulder muscles. There should be no pressure on the head or tension in the neck. The shoulders should be working hard and the breath should be steady.

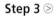

⊗ Step 4

Contract the abdominal muscles and, on an inhale, lift the feet from the floor, bending the knees. Move the feet toward the buttocks. The thighs should be close to the abdomen and the hips stacked over the shoulders so the spine remains straight.

Step 5 ⊗

Slowly exhale while reaching the feet directly upward until the legs are completely straight. The body should now be in one straight line. Lengthen through the whole body and avoid arching the lower back. Work the abdominal muscles hard to support the spine and keep the shoulder joints active and the chin parallel to the ground to avoid tension in the neck. Keep breathing steadily throughout.

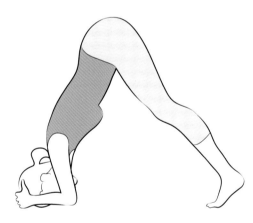

Headstand Pose

Shirshasana

During Headstand Pose, there is equal length through the front and back of the upper body, because it is in a neutral position, and the rectus abdominis and latissimus dorsi work to fixate the spine in this position. The elbows flex as the biceps brachii shorten and the triceps lengthen. The deltoids are in a concentric contraction and work in synergy with the rotator cuff muscle groups. The upper and lower trapezius and rhomboid muscles contract to depress and then retract the scapulae, creating support for the cervical spine. The gluteus maximus contract concentrically to extend the legs away from the pelvis, while the hip flexors, including the iliopsoas muscles, stabilize the hips. The quadriceps shorten concentrically, extending the knee joints, and the adductor muscles press the legs together. The feet are plantar flexed and the tibialis anterior is lengthened eccentrically.

muscle activity

prime mover

1   Gluteus maximus
2   Biceps brachii
3   Deltoids
4   Trapezius
5   Rhomboids
6   Adductors
7   Quadriceps

antagonist

8   Rectus abdominis
9   Latissimus dorsi

(5 beneath trapezius)

spine

The spine is in a neutral position and, therefore, does not move within a plane.
The pelvis is also in a neutral position.

Anatomy of the pose

Not visible from this view:

6   Adductors (inner thigh)

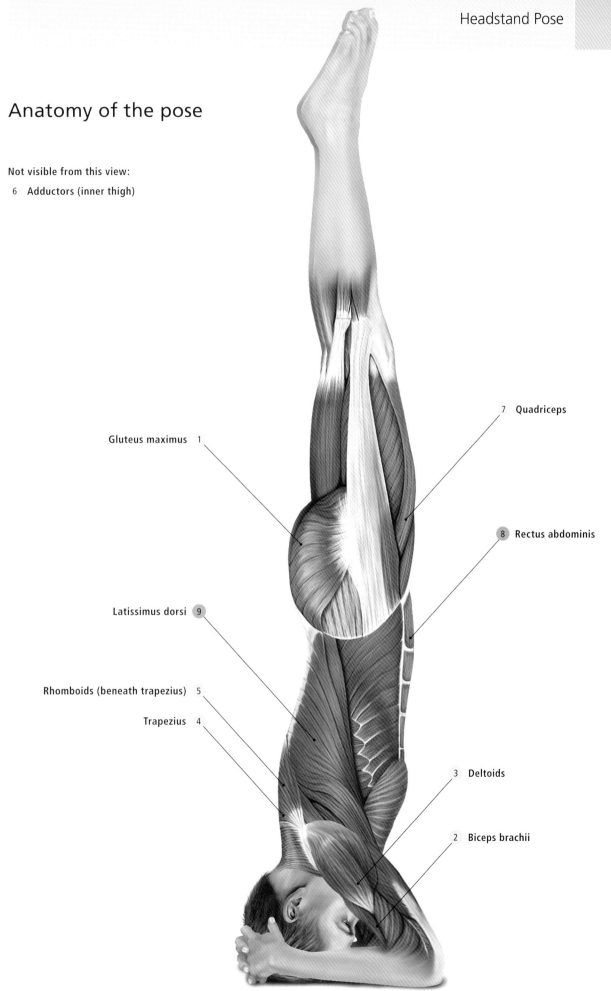

7   Quadriceps

Gluteus maximus   1

8   Rectus abdominis

Latissimus dorsi   9

Rhomboids (beneath trapezius)   5

Trapezius   4

3   Deltoids

2   Biceps brachii

Sequences

Yoga asanas can be linked together to form different yoga sequences. Variations of these sequences give us the many different styles of hatha yoga there are today. The classic Sun Salutation sequence is a good place to start when building up a practice of a yoga sequence, and there are many styles and levels of Sun Salutation to choose from. The following is taken from ashtanga yoga.

The first version is a modified version of the original ashtanga yoga Sun Salutation A, also known as Surya Namaskara A. This is generally repeated five times before moving on to another yoga sequence.

Modified Sun Salutation:

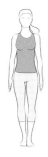

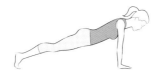

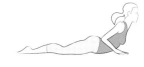

Step 1

Begin in Mountain Pose (page 54).

Inhale, reach the arms up overhead, and lift the gaze toward the hands.

Step 2

Exhale and fold forward into Standing Forward Bend (page 110).

Inhale and extend the spine away from the thighs, with the fingertips on the ground.

Step 3

Exhale and step the feet back into High Plank Pose (Kumbhakasana).

Inhale and rest the knees on the ground. Exhale and lower the upper body to the ground, so the body is now flat on the ground.

Step 4

Inhale and lift the upper spine into Cobra Pose (page 142).

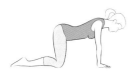

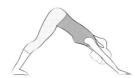

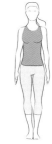

Step 5

Exhale and move into Box Position (page 55)

Step 6

Tuck the toes under and lift into Downward-Facing Dog Pose (page 164).

Step 7

Step the feet forward into Standing Forward Bend (page 110).

Step 8

Inhale and lift the upper body to standing, reaching the arms overhead before resting them by the side of the body in Mountain Pose (page 54).

Traditional Sun Salutation:

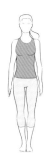

Step 1

Begin in Mountain Pose (page 54).

Inhale, reach the arms up overhead, and lift the gaze toward the hands.

Step 2

Exhale and fold forward into Standing Forward Bend (page 110).

Inhale and extend the spine away from the thighs, with the fingertips on the ground.

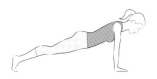

Step 3

Exhale and jump the feet back into High Plank Pose (Kumbhakasana).

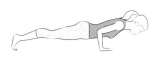

Step 4

Keep exhaling and lower the body to Four-Limb Staff Pose (Chaturanga).

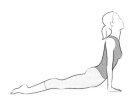

Step 5

Inhale and lift the upper spine into Upward-Facing Dog Pose (page 146).

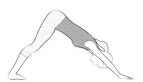

Step 6

Exhale, tuck the toes under, and lift into Downward-Facing Dog Pose (page 164).

Step 7

Inhale and jump the feet forward. On an exhale, fold into Standing Forward Bend (page 110) .

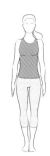

Step 8

Inhale and lift the upper body to standing, reaching the arms overhead. On an exhale, rest them by the side of the body in Mountain Pose (page 54).

Hip-Opening Sequence

By incorporating carefully selected asanas, sequences can be tailored to create different outcomes and to work particular areas of the body. A sequence that focuses on opening and stretching the hips would incorporate several asanas that gently stretch the quadriceps, adductors, hip flexors, and gluteal muscles. These movements would then prepare the hips for a deeper stretch, such as Cobbler's Pose (page 136), or Pigeon Pose (page 150) and help reduce the risk of injury.

The following is an example of asanas that can be linked into a hip-opening sequence:

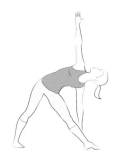

1. Triangle Pose (page 62)

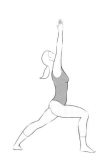

2. Warrior I Pose (page 70)

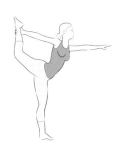

3. Dancer's Pose (page 96)

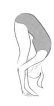

4. Standing Forward Bend (page 110)

5. Half Lord of the Fishes Pose (page 132)

6. Seated Forward Bend (page 124)

7. Cobbler's Pose (page 136)

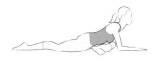

8. Pigeon Pose (page 150)

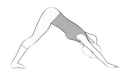

9. Downward-Facing Dog (page 164)

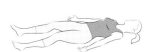

10. Corpse Pose (page 55)

Energizing Sequence

Sequences can also be assembled to challenge the body, for example, by incorporating asanas that move the spine into an extended position, such as in Wheel Pose. This invigorates the body and increases energy levels, partly because backbends release adrenaline, and so work well if the person's requirement is to stimulate the body and mind. An example of this kind of sequence is as follows:

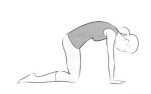
1. Cat Pose (page 158)

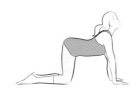
2. Cow Pose (page 158)

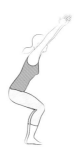
3. Chair Pose (page 58)

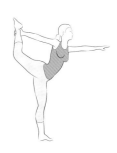
4. Dancer's Pose (page 96)

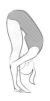
5. Standing Forward Bend (page 110)

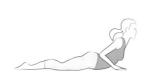
6. Cobra Pose (page 142)

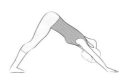
7. Downward-Facing Dog Pose (page 164)

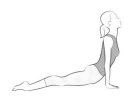
8. Upward-Facing Dog Pose (page 146)

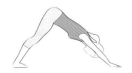
9. Downward-Facing Dog Pose (page 164)

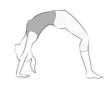
10. Wheel Pose (page 154)

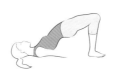
11. Shoulder Bridge Pose (page 168)

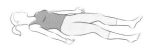
12. Corpse Pose (page 55)

Glossary

Abduction Movement of a limb away from the midline of the body.

Adduction Movement of a limb toward the midline of the body.

Antagonist A muscle that relaxes and lengthens while another, the "agonist," contracts.

Asana: The posture adopted during the practice of hatha yoga that brings about increased well-being.

Cartilaginous joint A slightly movable joint in which cartilage joins bones together.

Chakra The seven centers of energy within the body that align with areas of the spine.

Circumduction A circular movement of a limb extending from the joint at which the movement originates. Full circumduction allows for 360 degrees of movement.

Concentric contraction A type of muscle activity that results in the muscle contracting, or shortening, such as when a weight is lifted.

Depression Movement in a downward (inferior) direction, such as the shoulders moving down away from the head.

Dorsiflexion A type of movement (of the ankle or wrist) that causes the toes/fingers to move up toward the front of the ankle/wrist.

Eccentric contraction A type of muscle activity that results in the muscle lengthening, such as when a weight is lowered through a range of motion.

Elevation Movement in an upward (superior) direction, such as a shoulder shrug, during which the shoulders lift toward the head.

Extension A movement that increases the angle between two body parts. Extension at the elbow increases the angle between the upper arm and the forearm.

Fibrous joint A form of articulation in which the bones are connected by a fibrous tissue, mainly collagen.

Fixator A muscle that acts as a stabilizer of the body during movement of another part.

Flexion A movement that decreases the angle between two body parts. Flexion at the elbow decreases the angle between the upper arm and the forearm.

Frontal plane An imaginary vertical plane dividing the body into anterior (front) and posterior (back) portions.

Hatha yoga The system of yoga in which asanas are practiced for increased well-being.

Inversion A yoga asana in which the head is positioned lower than the heart.

Isometric contraction A type of muscle activity that results in no change in the length of the muscle, such as when pushing against an immovable object.

Lever A rigid structure that moves around an axis point when force is applied. For example, an arm is a lever and its axis point is the shoulder joint.

Planes of movement Used to describe movements of the body, referring to imaginary "planes" that divide the body into sections.

Plantarflexion The movement in which the toes and foot point away from the body, so that the angle between the foot and back of the leg is decreased.

Pranayama The practice of controlled breathing techniques used in yoga.

Prime mover A muscle that contracts to produce a movement. Also known as an **agonist**.

Range of movement The measurement of movement, measured in degrees, around a specific joint or body part.

Sagittal plane An imaginary vertical line running front to back, dividing the body into right and left. Also known as the **lateral plane**.

Synergist A muscle that assists other muscles to accomplish a movement.

Synovial joint A freely movable joint in which bony surfaces are covered by articular cartilage and are connected by a fibrous connective-tissue capsule lined with a synovial membrane.

Transverse plane An imaginary plane that divides the body into superior (upper) and inferior (lower) sections. Also known as the **horizontal** or **axial plane**.

Index